TEACHING THE
CHILD ON THE
TRAUMA CONTINUUM

TEACHING THE CHILD ON THE TRAUMA CONTINUUM

BETSY DE THIERRY

The right of Betsy de Thierry to be identified as
the author of this work has been asserted by her in
accordance with Section 78 of the Copyright, Designs
and Patents Act 1988

This book is published by
Grosvenor House Publishing Ltd
28–30 High Street, Guildford, Surrey, GU1 3EL
www.grosvenorhousepublishing.co.uk

A CIP record for this book is available from
the British Library.

ISBN 978-1-78148-449-4

TO THE CHILDREN AND
YOUNG PEOPLE WHO HAVE
BEEN MISUNDERSTOOD
BY ADULTS

CONTENTS

PREFACE

I have written this book because I am committed to trying to help and support the amazing job that teachers do. I have endeavoured to write in a style that is easy to read, with enough information to provide evidence to support what I am suggesting, but not too much that might distract from the main points. I have attempted to make it simple, short and to the point, so that it doesn't add additional stress to your workload!

In 1992 I distinctly remember a trainee teacher placement in Devon, where I was asked to pursue a five-year-old boy who had run out of the classroom and up a staircase which led to several different floors. After a thirty-minute panic running around a large Victorian school, I eventually found him hiding behind the coats and bags in a cloakroom. His tiny frame was shaking, and the frustration that I felt, and which was about to topple out of my mouth, was stopped when I looked at him and questioned what had happened to this little chap to make him respond in this manner. This incident was over twenty years ago, at the start of my journey of learning about children and how to help them recover from trauma.

This book explores the founding principles and philosophy that I have formulated for those who work at the Trauma Recovery Centre (TRC). The TRC is a charity that I founded in 2011 to bring together the wisdom of different professionals to work with children and facilitate their recovery and also that of their families. Our multi-disciplinary team of art therapists, music therapists, play therapists, creative therapists, psychotherapists, counsellors, social workers, teachers, teaching assistants and other specialists, are dedicated to supporting those children who are most in need of specialist trauma recovery help. We have expanded our charity while still specialising in complex trauma, and now provide services in two cities, with several more centres planned.

Having worked in a relevant field for 20 years, I have conducted my own research and developed theories which evidence the importance of effective communication regarding trauma for both the children experiencing trauma, and professionals interacting with these children. This has led me to write this book to collate the tried and tested methods into one place which focuses on exploring the impact of trauma on children and young people. I use examples of children whom I have worked with as a psychotherapist, but in each story the details have been changed to ensure their anonymity.

We are passionate that schools, police forces, social workers, lawyers, judges and in fact everyone who works with children, should have a working knowledge of the impact that trauma can have on a child or young person, in order that their recovery can be prioritised.

Thank you for taking the time to read this book.

Betsy de Thierry

MA Psychology and Counselling practice; B.Ed. (Hons.) Primary; Dip. Couns.; Dip. Life Coach; PGDip Play Therapy.

RECOMMENDATIONS

"This excellent book explains the continuum of trauma clearly in all its complexity in succinct and straightforward terms, drawing on the latest thinking and research in neuroscience. It shows how teachers, while not specialist mental health professionals, can provide skilled and effective help within school and the classroom to children and young people for them to recover from trauma. It recognises the pressure on teachers and schools to meet national educational objectives, which can all too easily ignore the particular history and personal needs of individual pupils. The knowledge and skills within this book will enable the busiest teachers to both recognise and to effectively respond to these particular needs, and of equal importance to develop their own skills in reflection and shared learning."

Bill McKitterick

Former Director of Social Care, Social Worker and Author

Bill has been a social worker for over 40 years, is the former director of social services for Bristol and author of 'Supervision', a social work pocket book published by the Open University Press. He now works with a particular focus on reflective practice and self-leadership in multi-disciplinary settings and his next book 'Self-Leadership in Social Work', is due out in March 2015, published by the Policy Press.

"This book acts as a useful guide to teachers faced with the often difficult task of identifying traumatised behaviour in school children of all ages amid the hurly burly of the working week. Betsy de Thierry encourages us to look beyond symptoms to understand more of what is going on. A working knowledge of attachment processes and of trauma theory, together with a focus on reflective practice, helps us determine what emotional scaffolding is required to meet the needs and aspirations of traumatised pupils in a holistic way. The book covers topics clearly and concisely and offers practical advice on management in the school setting.According to renowned child psychotherapist Violet Oaklander:

"All children are born with the capacity to develop and use all of the aspects of the organism [self] to live healthy, productive, joyful lives. We know that trauma interrupts the healthy development of the child. There are also some very basic developmental aspects that can further thwart healthy development. An understanding of these hindrances is the first step toward helping children heal."

A central tenet from Gestalt therapy holds that vital personal changes happen paradoxically when we embrace and accept who we are, here and now. When teachers respond in this way towards traumatised children, with clarity, empathy and respect, within the context of a safe, supportive school setting, this helps immeasurably. Such children may begin to develop the resilience they need to survive the vicissitudes of everyday life, in the classroom, the playground or at home."

Jon Blend

Child and Adolescent Gestalt & Integrative Psychotherapist

Jon works and supervises in private practice in West London. A guest trainer with the Oaklander Foundation www.vsof.org he has worked with children and families for three decades, mostly in the fields of NHS mental health. His chapter, " Am I Bovvered? " features in Relational Child, Relational Brain: Development and Therapy in Childhood & Adolescence (2011), Lee R and Harris N (eds.) pub. Taylor & Francis

"This book is an essential read for those teachers struggling to understand their role with traumatised children. In an easy to read style, it informs the educator about the neuroscience and psychology of trauma and provides practical classroom based tools to settle misunderstood, trauma based child behaviour. This book sets the standard for trauma informed care in the classroom!"

Julie Crabtree

Psychologist and Author

Julie has been a registered psychologist for over 26 years and has extensive experience in working with complex issues, trauma, and health. She is currently completing her PhD in the area of creativity and mental health and has authored 'Living with a Creative Mind' published by Zebra Collective.

"'Teaching the Child on the Trauma Continuum' is an extremely useful resource to support teachers in providing effective holistic education for students who have experienced trauma at any level. Insightful points are made about the impacts that trauma may have on the behaviours of students and the reasons for this from the fields of psychotherapy and neuroscience in an accessible and easily applicable way".

Paul Clark

Assistant Head Teacher

Paul has been teaching in secondary education for ten years, initially as a Dance Specialist and is currently working as an Assistant Head Teacher in Wiltshire, where he leads on the quality of teaching across the school. Paul frequently leads training both at school and in other contexts and is currently a Specialist Leader of Education appointed by the National College of Teaching and Leadership. Paul is passionate about high quality educational experiences for all students which take account of their differing needs and promote the development of each child as an individual.

"'Teaching the Child on the Trauma Continuum' affirms the role of teachers (and other school staff) as 'influencers' of children and demonstrates empathy and understanding for the pressures and tensions that teachers face. Betsy de Thierry recognises the anxiety that working with children who seem unable to access learning can cause and suggests a holistic ideal for working with them in school. Betsy's focus is on equipping staff and recovery for the children who have experienced trauma. Teaching the Child on the Trauma Continuum provides an easily accessible theoretical background to heighten understanding, whilst also offering numerous tried and tested suggestions for simple, low cost strategies to enable teachers and other school staff to effectively support children who have experienced trauma, whilst also minimising class disruption and teacher stress".

Annie Sempill

Social worker

Annie has worked in child protection as a community and hospital social worker with Bristol City Council, has been a supervising social worker for foster carers and recently she has become an independent social worker working in the locality offering specialist knowledge and support for families.

INTRODUCTION

THE EXTRAORDINARY ROLE OF A SCHOOL TEACHER

Teachers have the power to impact upon children's lives and change their destiny forever. A teacher is an influencer, a mentor, an inspiration, a role model and a caring adult who can look into children's eyes and speak words that change their lives.

It seems that the media rarely voices an understanding of the importance of a teacher's role or their relationship with children, but instead seems to be comfortable assigning to educational staff an increasing number of tasks and responsibilities that could be argued to constitute the parent's role. However, there is some literature available that recognises the importance of a positive teacher-child relationship, and Ginott movingly expresses the impact a teacher can have on a child's future:

> 'A teacher's response has crucial consequences... It creates a climate of compliance or defiance, a mood of contentment or contention, a desire to make amends or to take revenge. Teachers have the power

to affect a child's life for better or worse. A child becomes what he/ she experiences.

While parents possess the original key to their offspring's experience, teachers have a spare key. They too can open or close the minds and hearts of children.' (Ginott, 1975)

Yet what about that child who stares in silence and then replies with defiance, or runs out of lessons and then can't remember they even ran? What about the child who kicks out at everyone and everything for no apparent reason? Or the student who is unwashed, never arrives on time, and refuses to look you in the eye? What about the child with cuts on their arm? Or the one who is making themselves bleed as they pick at their scabs? Or the one selling herself to her peers and laughing boldly about it? What about the child who refuses to work, no matter how much you try to help them, because they believe that they are useless? Or the child who cannot sit still and seems distracted at all times? We've all had students that shocked us, worried us and frustrated us because they refused to engage in the class work that we had spent hours preparing, but what do we do? Surely we as teachers can't do any more?

I am writing this book as a qualified teacher and a child and adolescent psychotherapist, and it is designed to equip professionals who work in a school setting with an understanding of the impact that trauma has on children and their behaviour. It details the information that I wasn't given when I was a teacher, but instead had to search for, in order to understand the troubled children that I worked with. The first section of this book contains four chapters which explore how trauma can adversely affect a child's long-term future unless positive intervention is facilitated. It also looks at the core issues of positive attachment and building resilience. The second section consists of two chapters that explore children's responses to trauma. The third short section explores complex trauma and represents the small percentage of children in classrooms who can often create a disproportionate amount of stress for staff due to their volatility, aggression or lack of engagement. The final three chapters form the fourth section and offer some practical strategies for staff to use within a school setting. They also explore the role of the teacher as a key attachment figure. The last chapter offers some reflections concerning the apparent rise in secondary trauma amongst school teachers who work with troubled children and provides some suggestions to redress this issue. Through researching the effectiveness of the trauma recovery training courses for schools that I have delivered, I have found that this information does not increase teachers' already stretched workloads, but rather the evidence suggests that it decreases stress and secondary trauma, and actually increases job satisfaction (de Thierry, 2014).

It is recognised that 'trauma is perhaps the most avoided, ignored, belittled, denied, misunderstood, and untreated cause of human suffering' (Levine & Kline, 2007, p.3). This is the backdrop to this book and is a motivating factor to keep investing energy into facilitating appropriate changes in the culture of schools until the consequences of trauma on behaviour, emotions and learning are fully understood by the whole of society. Unprocessed trauma can lead to increased mental health difficulties during adulthood and a host of social problems, such as drug use, school failure, anti-social behaviour etc. It can also lead to neuropsychiatric problems, such as post-traumatic stress disorder (PTSD), conduct disorders, and dissociative disorders, whilst unprocessed trauma can also lead to medical challenges, such as asthma and heart disease (Perry & Szalavitz, 2011). When trauma is processed in the context of a warm and genuine relationship, the impact is minimalised if not altogether transformed into greater resilience, thus changing the trajectory of a child's life.

According to the Department for Education (2004), schools are one of the main potential sources of emotional well-being and resilience for children who have experienced trauma. Ignoring the problem seems not to be an option, following the publication of current statistics such as that one in ten young people are unable to 'cope with daily life' (BBC, 2013). Neuroscience can explain behaviour and trauma responses, and I believe that this knowledge must become part of contemporary teacher training, both in initial training and ongoing professional development.

I hope that this book will equip, inspire and encourage you in your role as a primary or secondary teacher. In the words of one dedicated teacher working in a secondary school:

> 'This book has provided invaluable and crucial information about the effects of trauma on brain development and the subsequent behavioural issues associated with this damage. This has ultimately had a life-changing effect on how I perceive, view and teach children in the educational environment.'
> (Rebecca, a secondary school teacher)

SECTION 1

FOUNDATIONS OF UNDERSTANDING TRAUMA

CHAPTER 1

UNDERSTANDING TRAUMA

CURRENT CONTEXT

The research suggests that there has been a rise in both the quantity of children affected by traumatic experiences and also the severity of the trauma experienced (Cafcass, 2009; Donnelly, 2013). These experiences have been shown to impact upon children's behaviour, their learning and self-regulation. In turn, this leads to an increase in stress for the teachers, who have to ensure that each child meets specific educational objectives that rarely take into account the individual history or context of each pupil. Consequently, stress levels are increasing, but there are a few key principles that can decrease stress and increase calm for both students and teachers.

Due to developments in neuroscience research over the last decade, there has been an increase in understanding of the concept of trauma amongst the general public. There are frequent commentaries in the media on the latest statistics regarding the traumatic experiences of children and young people, and it is thought that three children in every classroom have a diagnosable mental health disorder (Daniel, 2014).

THE TRAUMA CONTINUUM

Trauma is defined by Perry (2011) as 'a psychologically distressing event that is outside the range of usual human experience, often involving a sense of intense fear, terror and helplessness.' An alternative explanation is that:

> *'Trauma happens when any experience stuns us like a bolt out of the blue; it overwhelms us, leaving us altered and disconnected from our bodies. Any coping mechanisms we may have had are undermined, and we feel utterly helpless and hopeless. It is as if our legs are knocked out from under us.'* (Levine, 2006)

Trauma can impact a child's body, brain, memory, emotions, relationships, learning and behaviour.

Traumatic stress is caused by the exposure to, or witnessing of an extreme and potentially life-threatening event. Traumatic exposure may be brief in duration (e.g. an accident), or involve prolonged, repeated exposure (e.g. sexual abuse), with the former being referred to as 'Type I' trauma and the latter as 'Type II' trauma (Terr, 1991). Knowledge of traumatic stress, how it develops, presents, and affects the lives of those who suffer from it, may be the first step towards being able to interact positively with those affected by it. Teachers are responsible for the education of many children who exhibit symptoms of behavioural responses to Type I and Type II trauma, and yet are rarely equipped to understand what can escalate or decrease negative behaviour responses. Heide and Solomon (1999) have defined an additional category as 'Type III' trauma, which they propose is the type of traumatic experience that occurs when an individual experiences multiple, pervasive, violent events beginning at an early age and continuing over a long period of time. Evidence suggests that the experiences of many school children are represented by all three trauma categories.

Alongside the categorisation of Type I, II and III trauma, there is an increasing recognition of the consequences of interpersonal trauma, which is complex in nature due to the emotional involvement with other people, usually close family members, who have been passively or actively involved in a traumatic experience. Community disasters invariably provoke a degree of media coverage, sympathy and support. In such circumstances, recovery interventions for children, by the very nature of their being community-based, usually ensure that the relationships facilitate recovery. Verbal and emotional processing is natural when many individuals have witnessed or experienced a similar disaster, and such mutual support, care, expression of emotions and the ability to verbally process can facilitate a full and healthy recovery. However, for the victim, interpersonal trauma is difficult, if not impossible, to speak about and can cause an immense challenge for children who are dependent upon the very same adults who are mistreating them.

> 'The most pernicious trauma is deliberately inflicted in a relationship where the traumatised individual is dependent – at worst, in a parent-child relationship.' (Allen, 1995)

However, as a nation we have moved away from the silence surrounding abuse and today sexual abuse is beginning to be boldly reported by the media. There is now public exposure of complex family dynamics where children have disclosed abuse from their relatives. It has been the media's exposure of interpersonal trauma over the last decade that has increased public awareness of the concept and the associated problems. Such exposure has significantly benefitted advances in rigorous safeguarding as a norm and expectation when working with children and young people (Department for Education, 2004). However, there has been little discourse concerning the additional complexities of recovery from interpersonal trauma or complex trauma.

Traumatic experiences, and our responses to them, vary widely and therefore it is essential to use a trauma continuum (de Thierry, 2013) to describe how mild or severe a traumatic experience is. I have had conversations with various educational staff who say to me, 'all children these days are traumatised'; however, I would argue that all children know some stress, most will have experienced a crisis, and a large percentage will have endured a traumatic experience, but these would range in severity as shown on the trauma continuum. The trauma continuum can help all those who work with children to use a common language, which consequently enables a child to receive appropriate interventions that are suitable for their level of traumatic response. The trauma continuum is shown below:

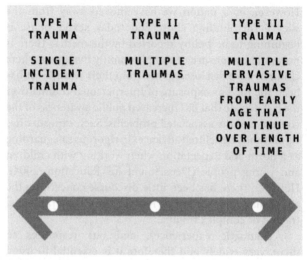

THE TRAUMA CONTINUUM
© Betsy de Thierry

The trauma continuum needs to be considered together with the parenting capacity continuum, which illustrates how great the impact of a traumatic experience may be. The parenting capacity continuum for the traumatised child is shown below:

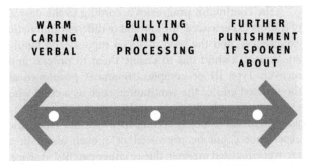

WARM CARING VERBAL **BULLYING AND NO PROCESSING** **FURTHER PUNISHMENT IF SPOKEN ABOUT**

THE PARENTING CAPACITY CONTINUUM
© Betsy de Thierry

A traumatic experience could be repeated bullying, bereavement, physical, sexual or emotional abuse, domestic violence or abuse, an accident, a severe illness requiring medical intervention, a parent's physical or mental illness, violence, neglect, etc.

The Type I or 'simple trauma' is usually defined as a one off traumatic incident or crisis. Simple trauma is difficult and painful and has the potential to cause injury to the child. This level of trauma usually has less stigma associated with the experience and therefore other people are often responsive and supportive to those who have experienced these traumatic incidents. This results in Type I trauma being placed at the beginning of the trauma continuum; especially if this is an experience within the context of a stable family where processing difficulties is a normal cultural expectation, as this could significantly limit the damage. For example, a car accident where the emergency services are involved but there is no long-term harm, or a child who has to adapt to their parents' divorce but this was handled with care, thereby limiting the emotional damage to the child.

The continuum progresses according to the degree of trauma experienced, the amount of different traumatic experiences, and the level of social support and family attachment a child has to enable them to process and recover. Type III or complex trauma is positioned at the furthest end of the continuum, such as a child who experiences multiple abuse and/or neglect over many years, without a family setting in which the traumatic experience could be processed or spoken about in a recovery-focused manner, due to either parents' absence, neglect or inability themselves to cope with the trauma. Complex trauma usually involves interpersonal violence, violation or threat and is often longer in duration. It is almost always an experience that causes a strong sense of shame due to community stigma, which can lead to the person feeling isolated and different. For example, sexual abuse, trafficking, torture, organized abuse or severe neglect.

Abuse and neglect in childhood affects a child's mind, their brain and its responses, their spirit and the ability to have hope, and their relationships with others.

THE IMPACT OF TRAUMA ON A CHILD

It is known that from early infancy through to adulthood, trauma can change how we perceive ourselves and the world around us, how we process information, and how we behave in response to our environment (Cozolino, 2006). Without appropriate intervention these altered cognitive processes and behavioural responses can lead to long-term problems, such as difficulties in learning, behaviour or self-regulation (Cattanach, 1992). When teachers are not educated about the impact of trauma on a child, then the needs of trauma victims can go unrecognised or are ignored, and the result can be that both students and teaching staff are unnecessarily stressed and experience further trauma.

Discussion Points:

1. What trauma experiences have your students experienced?

2. Where would they fit on the continuum?

3. What short-term response would you expect from that experience?

4. What long-term response could you expect?

5. What kind of life experience could place a child at the furthest end of the trauma continuum?

6. What level of the continuum are you confident and skilled to work at?

7. Can you think about a child who has been misunderstood due to their responses to trauma?

8. If you are working with children in the second half of the continuum, are you receiving regular supervision?

CHAPTER 2

RESPONSES TO TRAUMA – A QUICK LOOK AT THE BRAIN

Evidence has demonstrated that when the adults who work with children have an increased understanding of trauma, then it can immediately impact upon the life of a traumatised child (Alisic, 2012; O'Neill et al., 2010; Sitler, 2008). Basic neuroscience offers a simple overview of the neurobiological response to a traumatic experience, which can equip all professionals with an understanding of why children respond in certain ways. The human body and mind will display a predictable set of responses towards a threat or perceived threat, and having an understanding of this can reduce stress for everyone involved. The neurologist Maclean developed the Triune Brain Theory in the 1960s to increase understanding about how the brain is developed to respond to threat.

Maclean sees the brain as being in three parts: the pre-frontal cortex, the limbic, and the brainstem. The

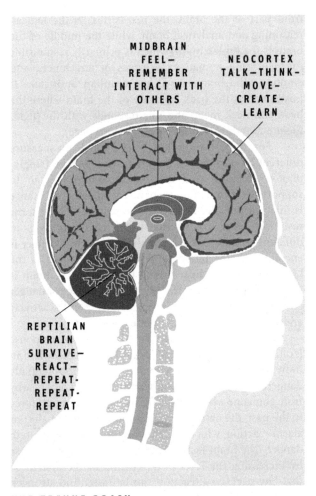

**MIDBRAIN
FEEL–
REMEMBER
INTERACT WITH
OTHERS**

**NEOCORTEX
TALK–THINK–
MOVE–
CREATE–
LEARN**

**REPTILIAN
BRAIN
SURVIVE–
REACT–
REPEAT-
REPEAT-
REPEAT**

THE TRIUNE BRAIN

front part of the brain, the neo-cortex, is the logical, reasoning and analytical brain, while the middle of the brain is the limbic brain, which is primarily responsible for managing human experiences of attachment and emotion. The brainstem is the reptilian brain and is positioned at the back and base of the brain where the head and neck meet, and this responds with the 'fight, flight and freeze' response (see previous page).

For some time it has been possible to measure different blood flows in the brain via a SPECT (single-photon emission computerised tomography) scan to support the triune brain theory. A radioactive substance is injected into the brain and the scan reveals patterns resulting from where the brain is responding to different stimuli. These scans show that when danger is encountered, the blood supply to the front part of the brain is reduced whilst that to the back of the brain is increased. This finding implies that in the face of danger and threat, the brain is designed to respond reactively and emotionally, rather than intelligently.

The initial stage of the fight, flight or freeze response is often called the 'alarm reaction'. This means that when an individual is confronted with a dangerous or potentially dangerous situation, such as hearing a raised voice nearby from someone who has been known to use physical force in the past, the natural brain response is a threat alert or alarm reaction, which switches on the body's reaction to danger. The brain facilitates this subconscious response by increasing the level of adrenaline in the system so that any necessary reaction can be faster and stronger, and it therefore becomes possible to run or fight. This primary neural activity occurring in the brainstem ensures survival, and leads to a significant reduction in the neural activity within the neo cortex, the thinking brain. The limbic area is responding via the amygdala, which is the emotional centre, acting like a smoke alarm alerting the body to the danger. When the threat is no longer present, the brain releases other chemicals to reduce the level of adrenaline. This whole process should be a time-limited response to threat in order to prevent the body from being in a constantly high state of alert.

The body's reaction to trauma is the same as the body's reaction to prolonged toxic levels of stress. Trauma or toxic stress occurs when a threat experience is so frightening

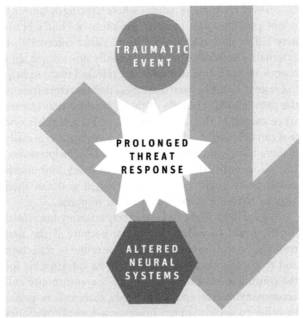

PROLONGED THREAT RESPONSE

that it causes a prolonged threat response, resulting in an altered neurobiological emotional state. A child who has an altered neurobiological emotional state, who is 'wired' to be almost consistently ready for threat, is a child who struggles to engage in learning. A child who has been hurt physically, sexually or verbally is 'wired' to remain in a self-protective defensive mode until the possibility of threat is diminished, even if the alarm response is reacting to a perceived threat rather than an actual threat, due to subconscious responses initiated by a previous trauma.

There are some situations where fighting or running is not possible, and in such situations a child's brain may aid in automatically freezing, either internally or externally. Automatic breathing usually slows down, and chemicals, such as endorphins, are released that can help to create stillness or even numbness that therefore lessens the pain felt. An example of this is a rabbit that freezes when caught in the car headlights, and is a familiar one that can be recognised as a response to trauma, especially if there have been previous experiences of helplessness. In milliseconds, the subconscious assesses how much power there could be to fight or flight and can then 'choose' to freeze as the only possible response.

These fight, flight and freeze responses are imprinted on the brain in order to survive, because if the first response to the onslaught of attack was one of reflection and reasoning, then the result could be catastrophic for the continuation of the species. The threat response and accompanying fear, enables a speedy, automatic response in order to avoid danger; however, when the response stays active for too long, it becomes toxic to the body and the mind.

PLASTICITY OF THE BRAIN

Only over recent decades has it become apparent that the brain has the capacity to change. Today, we are aware that different parts of the brain have different abilities to change, with the brainstem being the least malleable. A child's experience of life in their first five years is the most critical period of time for the brain to develop and change. The brain develops at speed, and the same plasticity that enables the brain to learn and change so rapidly is responsible for the critical damage when exposed to negative experiences during these early years.

In a child's first five years they relate to the world using their senses, and this causes the neurons to develop vital synaptic connections that grow their emotional and relational framework. It is again during these early years that the neural pathways are formed that create a child's expectation and intelligence. The more often an experience is repeated, the more likely it becomes a pathway and a set way of thinking and expectation. This means that if a child experiences abuse, neglect or unpredictable and erratic care, their brain is impacted and damaged. Children don't have the ability to choose to go for a run, find a therapist, buy a journal to write in or employ other helpful adult responses to trauma, and so are dependent upon those who care for them helping them to work out how to manage their feelings.

There remains a degree of brain plasticity for children, young people and adults that enables learning and changes of behaviour, but there is a greater ease in facilitating change and new learning during the younger years.

THE APPLICATION OF TRIUNE BRAIN THEORY IN A SCHOOL SETTING

When children feel calm and safe, they can focus their energy on learning. Children who are dealing with trauma are often in a chronic state of crisis and fear, and can be in a continual state of threat response; their focus is on trying to feel 'OK' or normal. When a child in a school setting feels threatened they will not be able to necessarily access their pre-frontal cortex in order to be able to negotiate, reason, evaluate or even think. Consequently these children can seem to behave instinctively without knowing why and can be triggered by seemingly minor issues. Their brains are so over activated in this way that they can struggle to learn new information or retain it for any length of time.

Another trauma response that is essential for teachers to understand is concerned with a traumatised person's ability to use words. When a person responds to trauma, the broca area of the brain, which is responsible for speech and language, goes 'off line' and shuts down. Therefore, to ask a child who just ran out of a class screaming, having punched another child, for an explanation of their behaviour *before* spending time calming them down, may result in them staring and looking blank, or responding aggressively because they can't access the area of their brain that is needed to use words. When a child reacts to a trauma trigger, it can be counterproductive to attempt to discuss the issue, because this adds stress and pressure to the child, who can be traumatised further, and also causes the adult to become frustrated. In fact, if the adult is aggressive in asking for logical reasons for challenging behaviour when a child has just exhibited a trauma response, the likelihood is that the child will become angry and their negative behaviour will escalate. The phrase 'speechless' is applicable to a person who has been traumatised, as the brain cannot access words to describe the experience, and it can sometimes take hours, weeks, months and even years for a person to add words to their emotional narrative of what took place.

TRIGGERS

Children can be triggered to respond as if they are in danger even when they are not, due to past traumatic experiences. Obvious triggers are when someone looks like a child's abuser or when the environment resembles, smells or sounds like the place where a person was mistreated. A child I worked with displayed strong emotional responses to fireworks, because in his subconscious they were the sounds of guns firing that he had heard as a young child. He was not cognitively aware of the link to his past in another nation, but as therapy progressed and he was able to make the connection, the crippling fear loosened it's grip. Donald Hebb (1949) wrote in his book 'The Organisation of Behaviour', that 'what fires together, wires together' and so often the triggers for a child which cause them to respond as if there is a threat, can seem illogical.

Robert's story can illustrate this subconscious reaction.

Ten-year-old Robert was walking his dog one day whilst drinking a banana milkshake, when suddenly a car crashed into the pavement and ran over his foot. A stranger called an ambulance and Robert was treated for a broken foot. In the lunch hall at school, many months later, Robert was happily getting his lunch and chatting to friends, when someone accidentally spilt their banana milkshake on him. Robert then screamed as if the car was crushing his foot again, flung his lunch tray onto the floor, curled into a ball and let out blood-curdling screams. After a teacher had reassured him, he stood up and felt overwhelmingly embarrassed, as he didn't understand that his subconscious was responding to implicit memories that still contain strong emotions. He knew he was safe and that there were no cars anywhere to be seen, yet Robert's response was one where his sensory memories, the smell of the banana milkshake, overruled his logical brain, causing him embarrassment. The only solution to this trauma response was to enable Robert to process his traumatic experience in the context of a safe, warm and consistent relationship.

Anyone who has experienced trauma can be triggered by any item that is linked in their subconscious to their trauma experience, and this can cause a threat response as if there is a real risk of danger or death. Common triggers are sensory related, for example sounds, sights, feelings and smells, or thoughts such as 'you're going to reject me'. In a school setting, a child who responds with a brainstem, survival response, by kicking, screaming, running or hiding, would often be expected to immediately discuss the reasons for their behaviour with a teacher. However, the usual cognitive abilities of the child would not be available due to the overwhelming response of the brainstem; their thinking, cognitive, intelligent, rational brain response is 'off line', as is their ability to access speech and language.

When adults understand that a child is unable to respond with rational, mature thinking from their pre-frontal cortex because their brain is still pumping chemicals that are responding to the threat, then they can respond with greater patience and empathy, which in turn helps a child feel safer and recover faster. **A child is rarely able to respond in a rational way when confronted with a perceived or real threat. Therefore, we as teachers need to change our expectation of them and utilise calming strategies as an essential relational intervention in advance of any cognitive discussion regarding their behaviour.**

When a child has processed their traumatic experience in the context of a positive relationship with an adult that they trust, they become able to regulate their emotional and neurobiological responses. This enables them to learn to stop just before the natural threat response, and sufficiently engage their thinking brain in order to be able to choose to adopt some calming strategies for themselves. This reflective response can develop naturally when a child is in an environment that is supportive and enables them to talk about their feelings, responses and thoughts in a non-judgemental

**COMPLEX
INTERNAL
SYSTEMS**

**TRAUMA
SYMPTOMS
AWARENESS**

**ATTACHMENT AWARENESS/
EMOTIONAL LITERACY
AWARENESS**

THE TRAUMA TRIANGLE
© Betsy de Thierry

way. A child can learn to self-regulate their responses when they have the provision of a warm, empathetic adult to help them process their trauma.

The responses to trauma can be conceptualised by using The Trauma Triangle (de Thierry, 2013) shown on the previous page.

The foundation level of the Trauma Recovery Triangle, 'attachment awareness/ emotional literacy awareness', suggests that opportunities and interventions for a child are offered which enable them to develop positive attachments and growth in their understanding of emotional literacy. For many children, any provision in schools facilitating emotional intelligence is a necessary addition to support those who have received inadequate coaching from carers regarding feelings, or who have had minimal positive attachment experiences. The emotional literacy skill set can also be effective for those children who have experienced traumatic difficulties.

The second layer of The Trauma Triangle, 'trauma symptoms awareness', is the suggestion that further interventions are required for children who are experiencing trauma symptoms. Two primary adaptive response patterns in the face of trauma are the hyperarousal continuum (defence – fight/flight) and the dissociative (hypoarousal) continuum (freeze and numbness). The position of self-regulation is within the 'window of tolerance', which allows for some hyperaroused and hypoaroused responses but within safe limits that enable an easy de-escalation to a calm place.

HYPERAROUSAL ZONE
HYPERVIGILANT
FLASHBACKS
EMOTIONAL REACTIVITY
AGITATED AND JUMPY
ALARM RESPONSE

WINDOW OF TOLERANCE

OPTIMAL AROUSAL ZONE

HYPOAROUSAL ZONE
NUMBING OF EMOTIONS
DISSOCIATIVE
SLOW AND LETHARGIC
GLAZED AND SLOW TO RESPOND
COMPLIANT
INATTENTIVE

THE WINDOW OF TOLERANCE
SIEGAL, 1999

Each of these response 'sets' activates a specific combination of neural systems, and in this second layer of the triangle, a child will potentially be responding with hyperarousal responses that are the symptoms of trauma (hyperarousal and hypoarousal will be explored further in Chapter 5). A child could be experiencing a single trauma symptom, such as sudden anger outbursts, or being continually agitated. If they are further along the trauma continuum, rising into the third part of the triangle, then a child may experience multiple trauma symptoms, such as flashbacks, nightmares, self-harming, and anger or compliance. With each additional adaptive coping mechanism, a child moves further along the continuum.

The third layer of the triangle, 'complex internal systems', is the complex trauma response. This is the internalised adaptation that enables a child to survive despite an overwhelming traumatic experience and unmet need.

A child usually needs to use both hyperarousal and hypoarousal adaptations to survive a danger or perceived danger. When a child is in a hypoaroused state, their trauma symptoms are not necessarily as obvious, as they are internalised adaptations. The invisibility of these adaptations could be essential to enable a child to continue in relationships with their abusers and therefore have some needs met despite the cost, but may also be due to the ongoing nature of the traumatic experience. Compliant behaviour is often unrecognised as a symptom of the traumatic experience of being controlled, in a state of terror and therefore not being able to vocalise or admit need, and yet this behaviour could mask a hidden internal adaptive survival response. Professionals will often assume that complex trauma would result from abuse, but it has now been recognised that neglect is just as damaging (Perry, 2006). Neglect can be described as anything that involves the failure to meet a child's physical, emotional, cognitive or relational needs. For example, there have been studies conducted where the effect of a lack of verbal communication or a lack of touch, such as cuddling, have been shown to have a significant negative impact on a child's brain, to the extent that the brain mass is smaller in size in a neglected child.

It is important to note that the standard assessment tool that is used with children, the SDQ (strengths and difficulties questionaire), *does not* identify complex trauma; therefore it can be common for the most traumatised children to miss out on therapeutic interventions as their SDQ score could present as lower than a child on the lower end of the trauma contiuum. It is also vital to note that the highly traumatised child's brain will not have the cognitive functioning capacity to process verbal and cognitive therapy approaches. They need creative therapies that are not dependant on verbal processing, in order to access the right brain implicit memory.

Complex trauma is the term used to describe these complicated and pervasive developmental and long-term consequences of the interpersonal victimisation of children, usually involving multiple events and prolonged exposure (Cook et al., 2005; Coutois, 2008; Luxenburg, Spinazzola & van der Kolk, 2001). It describes the dual problem of children's exposure to traumatic events and the impact of this exposure on immediate and long-term outcomes. Complex trauma outcomes refer to the range of clinical symptoms that appear after such exposures.

Trauma symptoms will be explored throughout the book and Chapter 6 provides an overview of these symptoms to enable the ability to identify when a child is behaving in a way that indicates a trauma history.

DIFFERENT APPROACHES FOR THE DIFFERENT LEVELS OF TRAUMA

The trauma continuum and trauma triangle are vital to help professionals working with a child to identify how traumatised they are, in order to then facilitate the safety of those children who are positioned at the upper end of the scale, because the intricacies of the complex trauma response require specialist intervention. Whilst emotional literacy and positive attachment experiences are a welcome addition to all children, those who have complex internal systems could find that many of the interventions provided to children at the lower end of the trauma continuum or triangle are counter-productive, and can actually increase their level of traumatisation. For example, a pop-up tent, which is becoming a standardised strategy for troubled children in primary school classrooms, could offer a secure, safe place for a child who occasionally de-regulates and becomes anxious or stressed. However, for a child who is experiencing the symptoms of complex trauma, a tent could be yet more individualised treatment that isolates, rather than facilitates their integration, and therefore reinforces the child's rejection and sense of shame.

One example of this was in a school that has embraced attachment knowledge and understands that some children require specialist care. A 5-year-old boy presented with challenging behaviour which was also causing significant distress to other pupils and staff. The school offered the child a teaching assistant to provide emotional literacy sessions and a therapist for 12 weeks, but when there was no change in behaviour, another therapist was suggested. This was a repeated pattern that resulted in the boy having four therapists before he was 6 years old. This caused his disorganised attachment style to be reinforced, as he assumed that all attachment relationships were short-term and therefore not wholly genuine. This child needed a specialised treatment plan rather than instructions on emotional literacy and more short-term attachment figures.

Sometimes we want to apply universal strategies to every child who shows signs of needing support, but a child who has been severely traumatised will require a specialised strategy plan for the classroom. The good news is that there are now advances in the understanding of complex trauma and effective treatment strategies, and so there are experts who can help these children recover in the context of a therapeutic relationship.

'We know now that their behaviours are not the result of moral failings or signs of lack of willpower or bad character – they are caused by actual changes in the brain. This vast increase in our

knowledge about the basic processes that underlie trauma has also opened up new possibilities to palliate or even reverse the damage. We can now develop methods and experiences that utilise the brain's own natural neuroplasticity to help survivors feel fully alive in the present and move on with their lives.' (Van der Kolk, 2014)

Recovery from trauma occurs best within the context of healing relationships.

Discussion Points:

1. What sort of things could trigger someone to respond to a threat response?

2. What is the priority for a child once they have exhibited a threat response?

3. Can you explain the phrase, 'what fires together, wires together'? How does that affect the behaviour of children?

4. Can you think of a pupil who has responded in an odd manner, and can you now reflect on what the possible reasons could have been for this behaviour?

CHAPTER 3

ATTACHMENT

To build a solid foundation for understanding a child's response to trauma, it is necessary to combine the wisdom of attachment theory, trauma theory and child development theory. The combination of these theories sets out a solid expectation of the normal development of a child's mind and body, which then sits alongside the understanding of a child's relational expectation as set by their first experiences of bonding or attachment with their caregivers. This is then framed by the understanding of the impact of trauma on a child's mind and body development and relationships.

It is clear from research that abuse, neglect and other interpersonal trauma have a significant impact on a child's attachment to their caregiver and that this then influences behaviour patterns that affect future relationships. If a child doesn't have the early experience of nurture and positive relational interactions in an attuned way, then their brains are unable to develop the pathways that are needed to engage in healthy relationships.

THE PRIMARY ATTACHMENT

A child is born relationally wired with a desire to attach to his or her caregiver, no matter who that person is, or how they may feel about the new arrival. This first relational attachment is designed to become the foundation of their sense of self, from which confidence and self-worth is found. When a child experiences consistent love, nurture and care, he or she then believes that they are worth that attention and are consequently able to trust others. It is now becoming widely accepted that the first five years of a child's life is the primary time in which the brain develops most significantly. The brainstem primarily develops in the womb before birth, whilst the limbic area of the brain is developed by the age of three or four years.

Levine and Kline (2006) explain that healthy infant development is all about the caregiver's 'attunement' or careful 'tuning in' to the baby's needs, and how the baby perceives the world as friendly or hostile depending on the quality of these earliest interactions.

> 'What is even more astounding is how this emotional growth between a mother and her newborn is the catalyst that 'turns on' the infant brain, releasing chemicals, proteins, enzymes, and other elements that actually shape both the structure and capacity of the brain'. (Levine and Kline, 2006)

This early experience of attachment begins in the womb and enables a child to form a 'secure base' from which to explore the world (Bowlby, 2006). A new-born baby will cry and screw up their little face until the mother begins to soothe and provide comfort; a baby responds with relief and the mother also sighs with relief. A father will gaze into his baby's eyes with love and wonder, and a baby will respond with coos and eyes that shine with delight in the repetitive, relational experience. The 'dance' between these two or three participants continues as a baby's needs are met, and a baby's brain forms neural pathways that then expect warm, genuine, kind and loving relationships. The practice of responding to the emotional cues of a child is called being 'attuned' to them and their needs.

When a baby cries there is increased neural activity in both the baby and the mother's brains, which lead to the connection response. This reciprocal response is the very essence of the positive attachment behaviour pattern between a baby and a parent, and consequently the neurons involved have been called 'mirror neurons' and were first discovered by Giamcomo Rizzolatti in the early 1990s. This has helped us to understand how humans can feel another person's feelings and respond accordingly: when a baby sees another baby cry, they often cry too; when a parent feeds their baby, they often open their mouths as their baby opens their mouth to be fed; and when someone sees a chair fall from a table onto someone else's head, it is not unusual to see them also wince as if the chair was going to harm them too. These examples describe the important role of the relational 'dance' between a caregiver and their baby, which should continue to develop throughout childhood. It is this process of attuned responding that establishes a reciprocal expectation system that then enables a child to learn emotional self-regulation during the early stages of development and to carry this through into adulthood.

In a violent or emotionally volatile home, the mother's stress levels would have an impact on the unborn baby who could then be born with higher cortisol levels before even taking their first breath. If a mother's stress continues and she feels predominantly overwhelmed, her baby's brain will be shaped for survival and defensiveness with an expectation of danger, even if no danger is present. A baby will then respond to this stress through behaviours such as agitation and restlessness, staring in silent fear, averting their gaze or moving in jerky and odd ways.

A child learns to regulate their psychological arousal because of the presence of this familiar attachment figure, who is able to respond in a repetitive and predictable way by either comforting or stimulating as needed. When an attachment figure is able to soothe the little one, it not only enables comfort at that particular moment, but it also enables the formation of a biological framework for dealing with future stress or need. The repetitive action of soothing and comforting a child when they are distressed enables the child to develop their own ability to rely on their own sense of security, thus creating emotional resilience. If a child doesn't have exposure to this attachment relationship of predictable, repetitive, calming, and soothing behaviour, they will struggle to learn to self-regulate their own emotions and will present with behaviour that reflects this status.

> *'The way that a mother treats her baby early in life literally affects which DNA gets transcribed and, therefore, the physiological path the baby's brain*

and body will take. This is where nature meets nurture. Here, nurture determines which natural potentials - positive and negative - will be realised and which will stay hidden in the double helix.'
(Perry and Szalavitz, 2010)

This primary attachment relationship hopefully remains with a child as they grow older and importantly, it also enables them to develop other attachment relationships. If a child hasn't had this primary attachment, it is challenging for them to develop other attachment relationships, as they haven't had the 'secure base' from which to explore the dynamics of a relationship.

Sadly, for many children this journey of security and self-worth is not a familiar one. For a significant number of children their primary caregiver is struggling themselves and so hasn't got the emotional ability to provide the consistency, predictability and nurture that a child needs to develop in a healthy way. Unhealthy generational behaviour patterns can be passed down that may be diametrically opposed to attunement and positive attachment, such as the 'stiff upper lip' culture which can be emotionally neglectful, or an abusive harsh family culture that produces fear and a lack of trust. There are many other family cultures that can be transferred to the next generation as expected behaviours and these can create entire family groups with similar dysfunctions that are then blamed on their genes.

> *Picture little Paul, who watches his brother work hard yet receive little affirmation from their mother for his successes, only constant criticism. Paul decides to work even harder to avoid the criticism coming his way, but when he is not affirmed at all, but is rather hit and screamed at, he gives up and becomes a school refuser. Similarly, little Jane runs to mum who took her to the park and played with her yesterday, but today finds mum is drunk and shouting at her. Sarah's father adores her and seems attentive and attuned to her needs, but he is also secretly abusing her and threatens to kill her mum if she tells anyone. These experiences are confusing for a child, because the very person they are drawn towards is the same person who is hurting them. Their experience of these early attachments will change every future relationship that they go on to form.*

When a child experiences continual inconsistency and confusion in parental responses, they cannot rely on their attachment figure to be a safe and secure base, and so their capacity for resilience and social confidence can be significantly reduced.

EMOTIONAL LITERACY

Not only is this primary attachment figure the 'safe base' for a child because they are the source of safety and comfort, but it is also within this attachment relationship that a child first learns emotional literacy. As the caregiver responds to a child's needs and feelings, they are also able to provide words to them. For example, if a child was crying after falling over and a parent comforts them and says; 'Oh dear, it can feel so scary when you hurt yourself, can't it? I am wondering if you feel sad or scared or upset right now?' Then this builds the child's capacity for reflective thinking and helps them to explore different words for different feelings.

When a child has not had these repetitive experiences in early childhood, they can find it unknown and challenging to be asked to reflect on or name any feelings that they may be experiencing. They will be unfamiliar with managing strong emotions and potentially have a fear of the powerlessness of such responses themselves. This uncertainty and inability to reflect upon or understand familiar feelings can lead to children using only behaviours to express their feelings. This can then lead to difficult relational experiences due to these expressions of strong feelings, which in turn can reinforce the fear and lack of trust within relationships. A child is already in a negative relational behaviour pattern that will continue into adulthood unless there is a person who provides a positive, consistent, predictable relationship, and spends time helping a child to learn these vital skills.

When a child experiences a repetitive negative response to their expression of need or feelings, then they will learn to survive with different maladaptive coping mechanisms. A story about Miranda can illustrate this:

Miranda is shopping with her mother, who is in a hurry to buy food before the school run when she has to pick up her sister. Mum is rushing around the aisles when Miranda slips over and screams in distress. Her mum is able to bend down and pick up her little girl, whilst offering soothing words with calming tones, 'Oh little one, are you OK? Oh dear, let's see where you hurt yourself. Oh dear...It's going to be OK sweetie.' Soon, Miranda stops sobbing and is happily carried on her mother's hip while she finishes the shopping and they get to her sister's school just in time to pick her up. The alternative version is where Mum is already emotionally overwhelmed, and so when Miranda trips over and screams in distress, she shouts at her loudly over the noise saying, 'Don't you know how late we are? Stop crying now or I'll smack you and then you'll be really crying. Come on or I'll leave you behind here on your own.' Mum drags Miranda along whilst mumbling nasty words about her daughter's inability to keep up with her.

Both versions of Mum are stressed and in a hurry, but one is able to offer a calm and soothing experience to her daughter, despite the hurry, whilst the other responds with her own needs and fears as the primary concern. When a parent's own emotional needs are too dominating, their child's needs cannot be met and this can also lead to a child having difficulties learning to regulate their own emotions. However, if a child experiences caring, relational interactions that are continually repeated and repeated, then they are able to trust that relational process and consequently have the emotional resilience to explore more relationships and new situations.

Resilience is actually created when children experience some degree of stress, but the fear or anxiety that they feel is then relieved due to the presence of a comforting, reassuring, secure adult. When a child experiences stress without such an adult being present, then they are aroused but with no skill-set available to be able to recover easily or manage their strong emotions.

ATTACHMENT THEORY

The first person to articulate attachment theory was John Bowlby, who coined the phrase 'the secure base'. His work was developed further by Mary Ainsworth in the 1970s, to help professionals who work with children understand how significant the early attachment experience of a child is. It was Ainsworth who defined attachment as consisting of two main categories: secure and insecure.

Attachment styles can be viewed as a continuum:

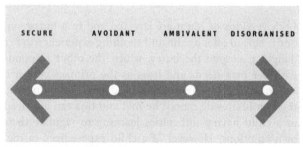

SECURE   AVOIDANT   AMBIVALENT   DISORGANISED

THE ATTACHMENT CONTINUUM

SECURE ATTACHMENT

A securely attached child is one who shows a good attachment to his/her mother and a sensible hesitation towards strangers. With securely attached children, their parents are available, perceptive and responsive to their child's needs, and are a 'secure base' from which to explore their world.

INSECURE AVOIDANT ATTACHMENT

Children with this attachment style do not naturally go towards their primary attachment figure whilst exploring, and show independence both physically and emotionally. When they are upset they do not seek comfort from their attachment figure primarily, which could be because they have had a caregiver who has been inattentive or unresponsive to their needs. They do not form friendships naturally and feel safe when in control; they are self-reliant and can have low self-esteem.

INSECURE AMBIVALENT ATTACHMENT (OR RESISTANT ATTACHMENT)

This is an attachment style that demonstrates ambivalence towards their attachment figure. Sometimes a child will be clingy, whilst at other times they struggle to be independent. They do not receive their security from their main caregiver and can be difficult to soothe when distressed. They can be aggressive and destructive, yet also clingy but rejecting when they get too close. This behaviour results from an inconsistent level of response to their needs from their primary caregiver.

DISORGANISED ATTACHMENT

Disorganised attachment occurs when a primary caregiver has been unable to be consistent and predictable, and has left a child confused regarding their needs. Sometimes the caregiver is present, engaged and loving, and at other times they are angry, volatile, rejecting, unengaged, abusive or inattentive. In such home environments a child does not know how to predict the behaviour of their caregiver and so they often need to remain in a defensive, threat response mode in case of further mistreatment, neglect or abuse, and they then have to come up with methods of coping with this confusion. Weiland (2011) describes the relationship between a child and their mother that can lead to disorganised attachment:

> *'The mother within this classification does, at times, provide caretaking and comfort. At those moments, however, this mother becomes very needy and uses the child to comfort herself – and so the child experiences the mother as needing comfort and the self as the comforter. The disorganised attachment mother may directly hurt or frighten the child...As a result, the child's internal working model (Bowlby, 1971) holds multiple senses of mother ('mother' being the child's earliest representation of the world): comforter, needing comfort, frightening or hurtful, frightened or hurt...'*

It's this attachment style that often leads to the most

complex trauma responses that take up a disproportionate amount of time for school pastoral staff. In Chapter 7 this attachment style will be explored further, alongside the trauma symptoms that often accompany it.

HOW THIS AFFECTS TEACHER – STUDENT DYNAMICS

It is common for children to project onto their teachers their subconscious understanding of adults and to expect them to behave in the same way as those who have been their carers. This projection is similar to the experience of transference, whereby a student transfers their feelings onto their teacher as a way of coping with difficult feelings about themselves. If they feel bad about themselves, they want to tell or show their teacher that they are bad. A child's attachment relationships will often be projected onto a teacher and this can create confusion within the classroom setting unless there is a clear realisation that the child does not usually have a personal viewpoint about an individual teacher, but rather is expressing a subconscious response to another adult.

When I train professionals about attachment as a foundation for understanding children's responses to trauma, I always notice a look of shock and anxiety as those who are parents in the room instinctively reflect on their own failures. The good news is that children seem to become securely attached when there is 'good enough' availability and predictability (Winnicott, 1960). It is normal for there to be fluctuations in the provision of attention and awareness, but the damage seems to occur when there is neglect or abuse and chaotic family dynamics.

If you do see the signs of attachment difficulties in your own child, it is rarely too late to try to bring healing to the ruptured relationship by making a commitment to focus on the needs of your child and spend time investing in your relationship with them.

Discussion Points:

1. What behaviour creates a positive attachment pattern for a child?

2. What parent/caregiver behaviour can cause a dysfunctional attachment pattern?

3. What are the main needs for a child to develop healthily?

4. How does a child learn to self-regulate?

5. Can you think of a student who shows attachment needs and what are you currently able to do to support them?

CHAPTER 4

RESILIENCE – HOW SOME CHILDREN COPE BETTER WITH TRAUMA

Resilience is the ability to recover quickly from difficulties and it's something that adults can nurture in a child's life. Whilst parents or carers hold the primary role of facilitating a child's resilience, another adult, such as a teacher, can significantly influence and develop a child's ability to show strength in the face of difficulty. I have sometimes been aware that in my role as a teacher I have been able to see my positive words and encouragement act like water to a droopy plant. I have witnessed children begin to flourish and strengthen within a classroom atmosphere where all children are valued and all children have something significant to offer the world. Teachers can therefore help children to develop resilience and a strong sense of self in the face of adversity.

The world can sometimes seem to be a frightening place and children will hear news of tragedies, deaths, family breakdowns, abuse and disasters. Whilst we recognise that it is impossible to shield children completely from stress and difficulty, the important question surely has to be 'how do we enable children to develop an ability to use the challenges and difficulties as opportunities to grow from, rather than cause further distress or dysfunction?'

The journey towards resilience begins at birth with the primary relationships or attachments whereby a child has a sense of belonging and security. The primary factor in building resilience is found in these repetitive, predictable, secure attachment relationships that a child experiences. It is in the context of these relationships that a child is enabled to find the skills of self-regulation and security in the face of trauma. Alongside these important life-giving attachment relationships where a child experiences the essential love, care, nurture and acceptance, there are other factors that can build a healthy resilience in order to be able to withstand the challenges of life.

I have developed the acronym RESPIRE (©de Thierry, 2014) to help others to remember the seven essential components in helping children build resilience. These key factors are: Relationships; Empathy; Strengths and weaknesses; Processing life together; Inner confidence; Responsibility; and Empowerment to make a difference.

RELATIONSHIPS ARE CENTRAL

When a child grows up in the context of a loving family, where they are celebrated, valued and have a sense of belonging, then they are more likely to develop healthy self-esteem and resilience.

When a child has a social system that provides stimulating relationships that are secure, warm, engaging, empathetic experiences, then they will be more able to grow up with the practised ability to reproduce more healthy relationships.

When a child is helped to form good friendships, where the skills of negotiation and sharing are practised, then they become able to be confident socially, extend their relationships, and explore their identity within this context.

EMPATHY FOR OTHERS

Helping a child to understand how others feel and develop empathy is a key skill. When they learn to value relationships, recognise people as individuals, enjoy their community and see themselves as a caring person, then they will become resilient in the face of troubles.

STRENGTHS AND WEAKNESSES

When a child is able to explore and determine their strengths and weaknesses without dread or a fear of failure, shame or disaster, then they will be more able to feel strength in their individual identity, and this will produce resilience in the face of challenge.

PROCESSING LIFE TOGETHER

When a child is able to discuss and verbally process emotional responses and see positive role models in the relationships around them, then they will be more able to be emotionally literate and articulate their feelings. This will facilitate their increased resilience in the face of difficulties, as they will be able to vocalise their needs.

When a child is helped to learn a musical instrument, become confident in a sport, or look after a pet, then they can be better able to self-regulate strong feelings through these 'hobbies', as both music and sport release endorphins which counteract the stress hormone cortisol. Having an interest in an activity such as sports, arts or a pet can help a child to self-regulate.

INNER CONFIDENCE

When a child is praised for demonstrating good qualities, such as fairness and compassion for others, and when they are affirmed for any other specific achievements this increases their inner confidence.

When a child has access to education and is able to enjoy learning rather than being pre-occupied with survival, then they have an increased chance of building resilience and building a healthy sense of identity.

When a child knows that they have a right to personal space and privacy, and they have a right to their own body, then they are empowered to not have to please the adults around them but instead can say 'no' to kisses, lap sitting and other unwanted attention.

RESPONSIBILITY

When a child has had a healthy attachment figure to develop a healthy sense of self, then they can understand that they hold some responsibility for their own responses and choices, and the resulting consequences. This becomes possible after they have experienced consistent nurture, care, love and protection from an adult, as a child will then be able to realise that they can try and learn some skills that could enable them to heal, get strong and build resilience.

EMPOWERED TO MAKE A DIFFERENCE

When a child is able to make a difference to another person's life and recognises that they can make the world a better place, they feel less powerless and more motivated.

When they understand their subjective life experience in context to other peoples' experiences around the world and are modelled generosity and compassion by adults rather than total consumerism, then they will develop greater resilience to challenges.

DEVELOPING RESILIENCE

A child that grows up with at least some of these experiences that develop resilience will increase their probability of having a greater ability to cope with the challenges and difficulties that arise throughout life. Resilience is built when a child has had some of these seven RESPIRE elements as part of a positive life that enables them to feel less overwhelmed and less helpless when a stressor presents. Schools can facilitate many of these experiences and already do, and they can help develop a child's ability to cope with traumatic events.

Trauma recovery takes place in the context of positive, warm, empathetic relationships.

Discussion Points:

1. What can be done to help a child build a sense of resilience?

2. Why do some children respond to trauma with a greater sense of courage and resilience than others?

3. Can you think of a student who needs to build resilience? What could you to help them?

SECTION 2

TRAUMA RESPONSE

CHAPTER 5

HYPERVIGILANCE AND MEMORY

Research evidence suggests that the building blocks of the brain develop from the bottom to the top (Perry, 2006). When children feel safe and nurtured, they spend more time in the upper building blocks of the brain where they do their most important learning, such as learning to communicate, getting along with others, reflective and logical thinking. When children feel unsafe or threatened, they spend more time in the lower building blocks of the brain, focusing on survival. When a child is unable to feel safe in the classroom, this can lead to changes in the brain that can include difficulties with focusing and paying attention. Children who have experienced trauma are often unable to feel safe and can be easily overwhelmed by minor stressors that other students may not even notice, such as the teacher being a little stressed or distracted. What other pupils may perceive as ordinary stress, a traumatised child may see as a life and death situation. This then leads them to an increased arousal state, which results in agitation or withdrawn behaviour.

AFFECT DYSREGULATION

The ability to regulate our emotions and responses is created during the early years of life, and is sometimes known as 'affect regulation'. It is something that is developed through the attachment figure of an attuned and well-regulated caregiver (Schore, 1999). When a child who has experienced trauma is struggling to regulate their emotions, they can often be seen as defiant or difficult, but it is not their fault. Trauma reduces their capacity to regulate strong emotions unless it is processed in the context of a healthy relationship. It can lead to ongoing difficulties with agitation, anger, reduced thinking, and impulsive reactions. These reactions can be defined as either hyperaroused or hypoaroused and are the two primary adaptive response patterns in the face of threat. A hyperaroused state is usually the first reaction to trauma, when a child reacts in a hypervigilant, alarmed manner that stems from the fight or flight threat response. A hypoaroused state is when a child responds by shutting down because they feel overwhelmed and they appear disengaged, numb or seem to be in a daydream. Both are signs that a child feels unsafe and that they are responding to a perceived or real danger (see the hyperarousal and hypoarousal diagram presented in Chapter 2).

HYPERAROUSAL

When a child is being disruptive in a classroom, often the easiest answer is to place them on the front row or close to the teacher, where any distraction can be minimised. Whilst this is ideal in allowing the teacher to monitor any adverse behaviour exhibited by the disruptive child, it doesn't take into account the possible reason that a child may have for acting in an agitated state. It could be that the child is in a hypervigilant state because of trauma and they are therefore feeling anxious about the behaviour of other children around the classroom. After moving seats they may feel even more exposed to a potential threat because they can't watch the room for signs of danger when they are sitting in the front row. A child is often expending the majority of their energy on being in the survival mode and being ready for the next assault or disaster. Consequently, when they have their back to potential danger they have to either twist and turn to look at those behind them in order to check the facial responses and movements of the other students, or if they are forced to sit still and look to the front, then they will probably have to dissociate in some way.

A child is hypervigilant when they are feeling unsafe. This could be due to a lack of attachment care or to past or ongoing trauma experiences causing subconscious triggers or anxiety; they are on 'red alert' to be totally ready for anything to happen. For example, other students don't notice when a door slams, whereas a hypervigilant child would jump or look shocked and look around them, with the accompanying physical symptoms of anxiety, such as sweating or palpitations. When another child moves suddenly and no one else responds and instead continue with their work, a hypervigilant child would quickly respond by looking around them to check their surroundings for any potential danger. A child may even run to safety or hide under a table to shelter from an oncoming danger that no one else is aware of, but their subconscious warns them that it is probable. This would not be a reaction that they are able to explain cognitively, but is a response from their subconscious.

> 'Faces are explored for signs of disapproval.
> Regulatory systems become biased toward arousal
> and fear, priming our bodies to sacrifice well-being
> in order to stay on full alert at all times.' (Cozolino,
> 2006)

In order for a child who is hypervigilant to feel safe, they need to be able to have an easy escape option to counteract the fear of being trapped. They need to know that they are sitting in a place within the classroom where they only have to watch some of the room, rather than maintain a 360 degree view. A corner seat is ideal so that they only have to keep an eye on the movements in front of them, rather than also be observant of what is occurring behind their backs. A hypervigilant child needs to have strategies to enable them to calm themselves, which is only possible once their positioning has been rectified. Then they should be able to focus on calming themselves with sensory aids, such as textured small toys to fiddle with or strong smelling comforting cream or cloth. These sensory strategies help a child feel 'grounded' and less anxious and stressed.

Sometimes a child needs to undertake an activity that releases endorphins so that they have a reduction in the stress hormone adrenalin. This could be as simple as squeezing a stress ball or jumping up and down a few times. Although it should be noted that it is always best to suggest that the whole class joins in with such an activity so that a hypervigilant child doesn't feel shame and experience unwanted attention.

> '*In this hyperarousal state, all of the necessary developmental tasks for their age will be sacrificed for the elusive goal of safety. In a state of perpetual hyperarousal, these children are unable to learn new things, play co-operatively with age-mates or develop feelings of attachment and security with their new safe care giver...*' (Silberg, 2013)

A hypoaroused child is one who is internalising their coping mechanisms and is shutting down, daydreaming or dissociating. This will be explored in the next chapter at greater length.

MEMORY ISSUES

A frustration to every teacher is when a child looks blankly and says 'I didn't do it', even when there is clear evidence that they did. Usually this is the response of a child who knows that admitting that she or he has made a mistake or had an accident that would lead to consequences which make it worth risking lying. Sometimes however, when a child is traumatised and does not feel safe, what may appear to be a lie is actually not as straightforward as would be initially expected. We would like to believe that memory is formed in our brains like a good film, with every scene that we need to access easily and readily available. Sadly, memory is a little more complex and much of our memory is stored in our right hemisphere in an implicit manner. Whilst in normal circumstances we may hold a large amount of visual memory, our bodies also store memory as sensations without any accompanying words or pictures.

We are reminded of cosy winter experiences when we smell logs burning in the summer, or of that time our dog was found to be ill when we hear a specific song on the radio; our brains have a way of storing memory that enables us to suddenly remember events, people and places because of a smell, taste or feeling. In the same way, our body holds the ability to drive a car years after learning, often without the cognitive memory of what we were taught.

Trauma and toxic stress severely disrupt the way that a brain manages, remembers and processes the emotional aspects of experience. The main emotional impact of trauma is outside of the child's conscious awareness and so they can struggle to remember or speak about or reflect upon the experience without an appropriate intervention.

Trauma is stored in the body as implicit memory that bypasses logic or understanding. The role of the hippocampus is to facilitate the integration from implicit memory and to integrate it into an explicit narrative with the help of the amygdala, which holds the emotional memory. In normal circumstances memory is integrated into the constant flow of life experience; however, trauma stops the memory from being easily integrated. When a traumatic experience occurs, the broca area (responsible for speech and language) shuts down together with the thalamus, which helps to translate sensations. The brain stem and the limbic area then take over and release hormonal responses to the threat, with this level of arousal preventing the hippocampus and thalamus from processing the information for memory. Consequently, memories from traumatic experiences are left as disorganised and fragmented sensory, emotional, visual, body sensations, which are in pieces that are not joined in an order that makes sense. Often the tiny details of feelings, sensations and other senses are remembered perfectly, whilst the overall narrative can sometimes be confused.

There was a child who used to regularly run out of her school, and she would hide under the bushes outside the school grounds or in the toilets and cry. This little child had been regularly sexually abused from babyhood and had never been able to fight back or run away. These feelings were stored in her body and so anytime she felt trapped or fearful she would find herself running as fast as she could. After a short time of hiding she would realise that she had run and would feel incredible shame, as the action had not been undertaken as a result of cognitive thinking and making a decision. Sadly, the response of the teachers at the time was one of frustration and they would ask her for the reasons behind her behaviour, but she couldn't verbalise her feelings or the triggers, or even really remember what had happened. It all seemed vague to her and her memory was predominantly of the feeling of shame. The teaching staff wanted her to understand that this was unacceptable behaviour and they seemed unable to comprehend that she was not able to control her running need. We were able to advise that she needed to be given permission to run whenever her legs felt the response, but this should be to the reception area where she should stay until she felt safe. We agreed that the only thing that would happen as a consequence of running would be that her teacher would check with reception that she was OK and when she returned she would be greeted warmly with a subtle welcome back. After a period of doing this she no longer felt the need to run any more, as she was able to discharge this pent-up trauma body memory.

UNDERSTANDING THE BRAIN AND MEMORY

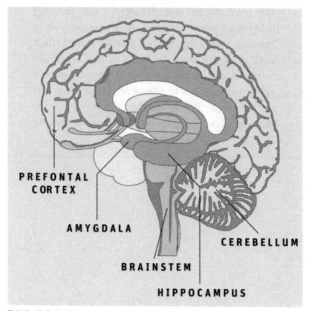

THE BRAIN

AMYGDALA – emotional centre
HIPPOCAMPUS – memory
PRE FRONTAL CORTEX – logical thinking
THALAMUS – interpretation of sensations
BRAINSTEM – threat response, breathing, temperature

Children who have suffered abuse or serious trauma may not be able to retain or be able to access explicit memories (left side of the brain, verbal) and may instead retain implicit memories (right side of the brain, physical, emotional memories) which do not have contextual detail. When these implicit memories arise, they can cause flashbacks, nightmares and other uncontrollable reactions, and these will be looked at in Chapter 7 together with other trauma symptoms.

When teachers confront traumatised children about their challenging behaviour, it is fully possible due to the responses of the brain during trauma and stress, that a child really is not able to remember what they just did. If a child has a trauma history and is in a hyper- or hypoaroused state, then they may well be so overwhelmed that immediately after a fight or incident they struggle to remember it clearly. This can cause problems within the school setting, but it should be acknowledged that during periods of high stress our ability to retain information is impaired and every person has a different coping adaptation which influences memory processing.

Traumatised children are lost in time because their past and present is mixed up and confused. They find it difficult to make sense of what has happened to them and they can feel confused about the intensity of their feelings and responses. Their memories are often a source of trauma to them and so consequently they can shut them down and avoid them. They need adults to help them remember aspects of their life and memories including any knowledge of their success and skills, as they find it difficult to own and hold onto these things. Positive adults can support these traumatised children by helping them when their memories fail.

'…trauma resides in our biology, not primarily in our psychology.' (Levine and Kline, 2006)

Discussion Points:

1. What behaviour responses can traumatised children demonstrate?

2. Why do they respond in this manner?

3. What can the teacher do to enable them to feel safe within the classroom and to minimalise the trauma responses?

4. How is memory stored?

CHAPTER 6

OTHER TRAUMA SYMPTOMS IN THE CLASSROOM

When exploring the possible symptoms of trauma that are present in a child at school, there are of course a diverse range, however, they predominantly fit into four major categories of childhood trauma symptoms:

1. A persistent fear state marked by primitive threat, alarm or survival responses, such as fight, flight or freeze.
2. Disorder of memory and trauma related memory disorganisation with flashbacks (intense memory recollection) and dissociation (sudden alteration in the integrative function of consciousness).
3. Dysregulation of affect and the inability to modify intense emotions.
4. Avoidance of intimacy and aversion to physical and emotional closeness that leads to feelings of vulnerability. (James, 1989)

This book has so far explored the threat, alarm response and how this presents within a classroom setting. Affect dysregulation has been explored, together with the importance of modelling self-regulation and reflective thinking. This chapter will attempt to paint a picture of the common trauma symptoms that may be observed in a school setting, namely flashbacks, depression, anxiety and panic attacks and self-harm. This is an extremely brief overview of the complex psychological difficulties, and as such should not be used in any way as a diagnostic or assessment tool, but merely as a rough indicator for education staff about the way some trauma symptoms could appear in the classroom. Ultimately, a child is only able to access the curriculum if they are able to be able to self-regulate and cope in the school context, and there are things that can be done to facilitate this.

The symptoms explored in this chapter are all identified within the Diagnostic and Statistical Manual of Mental Disorder – Fifth Edition (DSM-5), Trauma and Stressor Related Disorders, and can be found across the trauma continuum. The symptoms become intensified or there are multiple symptoms in complex trauma cases.

FLASHBACKS

Flashbacks seem to be misunderstood as memories that people choose to dwell on; the reality is that they are invasive, sudden, uncontrollable sensory memories that cause great distress because it seems like a traumatic experience is reoccurring. When a flashback takes place, the memories of past traumas that have been held in the body feel as if they are happening in the here and now. A person may see, smell or hear something that is a trigger to their subconscious memories of a traumatic event and this confuses the brain into believing that the experience is occurring again. Flashbacks are common for people who have experienced the shock of traumatic events and they are also a symptom of PTSD.

Flashbacks can affect children in the classroom and it is terrifying for a child as the memory can feel as if it came from nowhere. They cause deep distress and fear because it seems that they are not in control of the past. Sometimes a flashback is short and brief, but they can also be complex and cause strong bodily responses, such as fainting or screaming. A child needs to be reassured that whatever is scaring them is not happening now. They need to be calmed and comforted until they are able to access their pre-frontal cortex, the logical brain, and know that it is a past memory.

> 'Each time a [traumatised person] has a flashback or nightmare, or is merely startled by a sudden sound or movement, his heart, lungs, muscles, blood vessels, and immune system are primed to save his life - from nothing at all.' (Beaulieu, 2003)

ANXIETY AND PANIC ATTACKS

When a child feels anxious because of unprocessed trauma or because they feel unsafe due to ongoing difficulties, they may not be aware that what they are feeling in their body is related to their feelings of anxiety. A child rarely knows that they are feeling anxious until the definition is explained to them. Their body could express this anxiety in a number of ways:

- Heart pounds, races, skips a beat and chest feels tight or painful
- Tingling or numbness in toes or fingers
- Butterflies in the stomach
- Having to go to the toilet more often
- Feeling agitated or restless
- Tense muscles and body aching
- Sweating, dizzy, light-headed and shallow breathing

It is so important that children have some understanding of what anxiety feels like, so that they will be able to ask for the help that they need. When children experience symptoms of anxiety, these can often be compounded by a lack of understanding and an increase in fear about what they are experiencing. Often when children experience panic attacks, the anxiety they were feeling which led to the increased anxious state is compounded by the terror of the attack. They usually have no understanding of the nature of a panic attack and think that their increased heart rate, blood pressure and chest tightening are a heart attack and that they are dying. Obviously this is a terrifying experience for a child who is already struggling with fear. A simple biological explanation of the body's response to fear can help to stabilise a child and enable them to manage their anxiety until further help is offered.

DEPRESSION

When a child or young person is depressed, many changes may be observed. They may show signs such as:
- A loss of interest in activities that they used to enjoy
- Headaches or tummy pains

- A change with their relationship with food
- Feeling tired all the time, exhausted
- Struggling to remember things, concentrate or make decisions
- Self-harming behaviours or the expression of suicidal thoughts
- Disturbed sleep or sleeping far too much
- Little self-confidence
- Feelings of guilt for no reason
- Low mood, grumpy or irritable
- Socially withdrawn, bored
- Poor self-esteem
- Tearful
- Running away from home

Parents may not always be aware of depression in their children, and if a teacher thinks that a child may be depressed it can be invaluable to ask them how they are, when the rest of the class is distracted or has left the classroom. Even if a child may not use this opportunity to speak, they will know that you care and this is significant for their sense of worth and value.

SELF-HARM AND EATING DISORDERS

Self-harm is becoming increasingly common. However, it is a complex psychological response to a number of different powerful feelings, thoughts and experiences. If it is a trauma symptom rather than a brief adolescent experiment, a child may well have a sense of self-loathing that has been created through trauma. Children naturally blame themselves when things go wrong and this can lead to self-hatred if there is no intervention provided for a child, in order to process these feelings and understand that they were not to blame. When a child is abused they may feel a deep conflict between relief that they have been noticed and a terror and hatred of what has taken place. This conflict can lead to a sense of self-loathing which could lead to self-harming behaviours, be these eating- or cutting-related behaviours or more hidden self-harming addictions.

Sometimes children may become addicted to self-harming behaviours because of their need for the chemical response to their behaviour. Children often describe the experience of 'feeling alive' or 'feeling normal' when they cut themselves, as they struggle to lift themselves from a place of hypoarousal where everything becomes numb and glazed. The opioids that are released when hurting themselves can be addictive and can be a way of a child self-medicating to help them cope with the internal pain that they feel because of the trauma. When a child is desperate to break out of the internal chaos of a traumatised inner world, cutting can be a simple way of expressing their need and feeling relief. Sadly, many people mock cutting as an attention-seeking behaviour, but if a child's motivation is for attention, which is true in only a small percentage of cases, questions need to be asked about why they are feeling emotionally neglected and why they would go to these lengths to ask for help.

LYING AND MAKING UP STORIES

It is recognised that many children use lies and made-up stories to protect themselves from the reality of their own life experience. Lying can be a trauma symptom, and as such we would expect there to be a reduction of it during therapy or in a positive attachment relationship where a child can begin to feel safe enough to face the realities of their own trauma. It can be easier for a child to tell their teacher that their dog died or their car broke down as the reason for feeling upset than because they were abused or have witnessed domestic violence.

AGGRESSION AND IRRITABILITY

A familiar issue in a school setting is one of aggression and irritability. Aggression can be a fight response from the brainstem that bypasses logical thinking and this has been explored in chapter 2 as behaviour that could be due to a child feeling threatened and unsafe, and therefore responds with their brainstem because their neo cortex goes 'offline', preventing rational or logical thinking.

When a child feels continually stressed, hyperaroused and tense, they are unable to regulate their responses to triggers or additional stressors and may respond aggressively to stimuli as part of the 'fight response'. A child responds to an external or internal stimuli (a negative thought or experience) and this causes a subjective experience (feelings of sadness, fear or anger) which lead to a physiological response (usually increased heart rate) that triggers sudden behaviour (aggressive or avoidant). This emotional dysregulation creates behaviour that is over-reactive such as aggression, shouting, bursts of anger, crying or accusing.

When a child responds with aggression, the adult's approach that de-escalates the behaviour needs to be one of reflection rather than further anger and aggression. The child usually responds with surprise and warmth when an adult looks at the aggressive actions, and having restrained the child if necessary to stop anyone getting hurt, then comments, 'I wonder why you are responding like this. What could have caused you to feel such strong feelings?' This reflection can disarm a child's need to defend and can lead to them being able to calm themselves faster which then enables a discussion regarding the consequences of their actions.

THERE IS HOPE FOR CHILDREN WHO ARE WOUNDED THROUGH TRAUMA

Children begin to recover from their traumatic experiences when they are able to interact with a dependable, empathetic and warm adult who demonstrates care for them. Ideally, children need to have access to professional trauma therapy where they are able to have a therapeutic relationship, and also the time and space to process the trauma. A teacher and any additional education staff can also be significantly beneficial in helping children to experience more positive attachments that can facilitate them to develop increased self-esteem, confidence, an understanding of their own trauma responses, and self-regulation. This role is discussed further in the fourth section of this book.

> 'Therapeutic approaches must be directed at the areas of the brain which mediate this alarm-fear-terror continuum.' (Perry et al., 1993)

The holistic ideal would be that a parent also has parenting input that enables them to understand how trauma has affected them and their children in order to motivate them to focus on their recovery too. Ideally, teachers should communicate with therapists and any social workers or other services that are working with the family, so that recovery can be the focus for every professional. This model of a team around the child is essential for clear communication and clear objectives that are centred on recovery from trauma.

Through child-parent interactions and sensory play activities, neural connectors are increased and trauma-induced brain damage can be repaired. (Perry, 2004; Siegel, 2004).

Discussion Points:

1. What trauma symptoms have you seen in the classroom?

2. Did you think they were trauma symptoms or defiant/irritating behaviour and how has this changed?

3. Where would you refer a child who shows concerning behaviour?

SECTION 3

UNDERSTANDING COMPLEX TRAUMA – THE FURTHEST END OF THE TRAUMA CONTINUUM

CHAPTER 7

THE ULTIMATE OVERWHELMED TRAUMA RESPONSE

Complex trauma is misunderstood and often unrecognsied. The trauma contiuum is not usually articulated, thus leading to the most traumatised people not being understood or having their needs recognised, but instead being treated in a similar way to those who have endured short term, simple trauma. People who have experienced complex trauma have symptomology that is similar to PTSD although recognises the extensive duration of the traumatic experience. The DSM 5 has an extensive list of symptoms of PTSD, many of which are explored in this book; this chapter focuses on dissociation as a symptom that is often misdiagnosed and misunderstood

When working with children, I speak to them about there being two buckets inside all people: there is a shiny, sparkly bucket that has the purpose of collecting the love, affirmation and value that others give, and a muddy, dirty bucket that exists to contain all the nasty things that happen that are too difficult to deal with at the time. The shiny bucket gives a person a sense of worth and also builds inner strength to be able to be less deeply affected by traumatic experiences, whilst the muddy, dirty bucket is useful for the short-term ability to continue with a normal looking life and not have to be disrupted by the need to process emotional responses immediately. It can become necessary to pile up the mud and rubbish that is thrown in the bucket during the tough times of life, because when difficult things happen, the strong feelings of fear, anxiety or anger cannot always be held in conscious thoughts due to the need to remain functioning in a public setting. Therefore, this is an internal mechanism which enables these strong feelings to be 'stored' in a 'bucket' until there is time and space or the emotional courage to process them.

When there is a continual onslaught of difficult times and traumatic experiences, a child's bucket can become full. At this stage of emotional capacity they may find themselves emotionally leaking by finding that their attitudes are negative or that they are unable to concentrate due to the discomfort of the 'full bucket internally rumbling' as it demands attention. They could find themselves seeking short adrenaline highs that distract from the emotional pain of feeling full to capacity of strong emotion, and so they quickly pinch their neighbour or seek to subtly irritate another child during class. If difficulties continue, then it is possible that a child could even have an emotional explosion, due to a lack of ability to hold the bad experiences in. This explosion is a common scene in a school, for example when a child in a primary setting has a tantrum, with arms and legs flying, or in a secondary setting when they may find themselves exploding onto another person because of what seems to be a disproportionately small irritation.

As teachers we recognise that when our personal situations are challenging, these need to be emotionally set aside to focus on the school day. Hopefully, there is a common recognition about the importance of sharing these difficulties with others when possible so that the impact of them is minimalised and we too avoid 'leaking' onto others.

If a child has learned that the consequence of bad behaviour depletes the shiny internal bucket because they are reprimanded and feel bad, then they may find themselves having to create an alternative way of handling the strong feelings that are a result of negative experiences, and they may have to create another bucket. The same cycle can occur again and another bucket may be created, and so it continues until a complex internal system is created that has different buckets that hold different memories and experiences, and the feelings associated with them. This is called dissociation, and it is a way of separating and detaching from some of the traumatic experiences because of their overwhelming nature.

The type of traumatic experience that could lead to a child becoming dissociative could be interpersonal trauma, where the caregiver is also the main cause of trauma, or medical trauma, where there is severe intervention rendering a child powerless. Alternatively, it could be a community disaster, such as gang violence, war and natural disasters, or trauma involving family dynamics, such as parental loss or family chaos.

The definition of dissociation found at the Institute for the Study of Trauma and Dissociation (ISSTD) is as follows:

'In order to feel safe, the person needs to separate
the emotions, physical sensation or experiences
completely from her awareness so that she, outside
of conscious awareness 'creates' separate parts
of herself to hold these emotions, sensations or
experiences.' (ISSTD, 2009)

**Dissociation becomes an effective coping strategy
if fighting or escaping are not possible options,** as it
enables a traumatised person to cope with overwhelming
fear or helplessness. However, it can lead to an increase
in long-term challenges that can be highly damaging to
their personality, as it is a way of withdrawing from the
outside world to focus instead on the inner world in order
to survive. It should be noted that if a child is dissociative,
this does not mean that they are currently in a situation
where they are being mistreated. Dissociation usually
persists even if a child is safe and within a supportive
environment, and can continue until a child receives the
appropriate therapy.

Dissociative responses are also placed along a
continuum and begin as experiences that would be
familiar to everyone. For example, when we are driving
or absorbed in a film or a book, we may be somewhat
disconnected to the outside world as we focus on other
stimuli, and this causes our reactions to be slower to
other people and there may be a glazed or dreamy look.
Dysfunctional dissociation occurs to protect a child from
their experience and is problematic when they have no
control over the reaction. A mild dissociative response
would be when a child looks like they are in a trance or
'spaced out' and seems unaware of their surroundings,
whilst severe dissociation is when a child separates
completely from their experience.

Children can learn to 'switch off' their feelings when their bodies hurt too much from abuse or torture. Dissociation acts like an anaesthetic in the short term in order to protect a person from experiencing pain but can then become a behaviour pattern called 'depersonalisation'. This is when a child has blocked out the feelings in his or her body or other senses like hearing, seeing or tasting. Sometimes a child needs to escape from the traumatic experience but because they can't physically leave, they mentally separate instead. They can develop a skill called 'derealisation' whereby the present surroundings feel unreal.

> *For example, a little girl who is eight years old spoke proudly of having a hard body that doesn't feel any pain. She looked at me with a glowing face and said that she can't feel it when she is punched by bullies and can't feel any pain when anyone hurts her, ever. She explained that she has special magic dogs that are all over her skin on the inside and they destroy any feeling of pain. The problem is that whilst this depersonalisation helps her deal with the pain of the abuse, she is now struggling with encopresis because she is not confident in feeling anything below the waist.*

The most severe end of the dissociation continuum occurs when a child has to separate completely into fragmented parts, and this can cause chaos for a child when in the classroom setting.

'The most serious end of the dissociation continuum happens when the child, in order to escape the terrifying event, has to separate so completely from himself that it feels as if separate selves hold the awful feelings, thoughts and memories. These are called 'dissociative parts' (also referred to as 'dissociative states'), and mean that the child is still one individual but has separate parts of the self with separate awareness or 'consciousness'. These parts of the child's mind can hold the unwanted and unacceptable feelings, thoughts, and frightening memories away from the child's ongoing awareness so he doesn't need to experience them. Otherwise, it would be too hard for him to go about his daily life and do what is expected of him. This type of dissociation can be referred to as a disturbance or disruption in his identity (not a unified self): having separate parts or states of awareness rather than one state of awareness for all of the feelings, thoughts and behaviours.' (ISSDT, 2009)

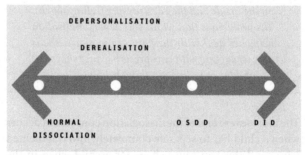

DEPERSONALISATION

DEREALISATION

NORMAL   O S D D   D I D
DISSOCIATION

OSDD = Other specified dissociative disorder
DID = Dissociative Identity Disorder

THE DISSOCIATIVE CONTINUUM

BEHAVIOUR IN THE CLASSROOM

To the teacher, a dissociative child may look like a normal child who has behaviour difficulties, such as marked and sudden behaviour changes that can conflict in presentation. However, a child may seem to lie about events or their behaviour because they have separate 'parts' that have no memory of the actions of the other.

Some dissociative behaviours can be disruptive to the whole class, or to the child's social experience and ability to engage in learning, or are disruptive to the staff. Typical behaviours are sudden changes in mood that are more significant and contrasting than normal, and a child presenting behaviours that seem to be differing in developmental age, such as acting as a needy pre-school child and then behaving as an eight-year-old child within the same hour. They may suddenly demand to use several names, and change their appearance, friends and favourite activities. A dissociative child changes from being hyperaroused to hypoaroused within a short space of time, and there are also changes in their social skills and learning levels on different days or in different lessons.

The disruptions to learning include the behaviour challenges but also involve difficulty in remembering significant events and experiences, whilst struggling to concentrate and focus at times, yet at other times being capable of intense concentration. Socially, they can find forming friendships challenging as they are not predictable themselves and can be withdrawn on one day, and be hyperaroused and aggressively extroverted another day.

A teacher rang me and with deep sighs explained the chaos that one eight-year-old boy called James was causing in her school. He was kicking, hitting and pinching other children, and was also shouting foul language at the teacher in front of the rest of the class. The problem was that James totally denied that he had done any of these things and couldn't seem to remember any incidents of bad behaviour. When he was being aggressive he seemed to regress to speaking and acting like a much younger child, but would then speak later with the staff in an articulate and well-mannered way, expressing his horror that anyone would behave in such a way in school. Sometimes he would be found in different places within the school building, shaking, crying and lying in a curled up position. When James was like this he seemed to be unaware of his surroundings and wouldn't be able to speak; he simply whined and whimpered but used no words. Again when the staff attempted to ask James what was happening to him when he was shaking and crying, he articulately denied such odd behaviour. I asked questions about James' past and it transpired that he had been adopted when he was three years old, and when with his birth family he had experienced severe neglect and abuse. I explained that the child seemed to be presenting with dissociative symptoms that would need appropriate specialist therapy treatment over several years. After two years of intense treatment with his therapist James made an excellent recovery and was able to excel at school.

THE DAISY THEORY (DE THIERRY, 2006)

This theory is one that I have developed in my work with children and families to explain the way that a dissociative child has learned to cope with their traumatising experience. As a starting point, it can be useful to grasp the concept of a healthy internal system using an image of a row of three peas with the letters 'V' for vulnerable, 'I' for inner child and 'P' for professional, to represent the three internal states that we all have. Many people live as a professional person, leading a fulfilling life whilst also having a vulnerable state that allows heartfelt responses, relationships, and deep values and beliefs. Whilst the vulnerable state influences the professional state, there is the ability to have separation. When these 'states' are combined with a healthy inner child that engages with play or recreation, this then results in a contented, fulfilled adult. Each person has a different size for each part, for example artists may struggle to live in a professional state, as they depend on their vulnerable state to produce meaningful art work, and yet high-flying business people may have a significantly smaller vulnerable state, as it is given little attention due to the primary focus of their energy.

As life becomes more complicated and new roles are taken on, new states may become apparent. These are not dissociative states, but merely different states of 'being'.

In the daisy diagram these different states are represented by the petals.

In line with a psychological theory called the Ego State Therapy Theory, by Watkins and Watkins, which is often referred to as the 'dissociation pie' model (1979, 1993), the petals are separated by thin lines that represent no dissociation, whereas thicker lines indicate that the separation becomes more significant and could be amnesic. In order to also include the structural dissociation theory of Van der Hart, Nijenhuis and Steele (2006), the middle of the daisy is often seen as the apparently normal part (ANP) or the presenting part, and the petals are seen as an emotional part (EP).

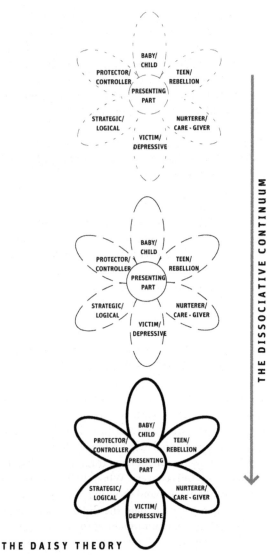

THE DAISY THEORY

© Betsy de Thierry

The daisy with the thick amnesic walls would be a person with dissociation identity disorder (DID), where the thickness of the walls enables them to continue to function although not as a whole integrated self. Previously, DID used to be called multiple personality disorder (MPD). The daisy model enables people to understand the dissociative continuum with ease.

> *'Trauma related structural dissociation then, is a deficiency in the cohesiveness and flexibility of the personality structure.'* (Van der Hart, Nijenhuis and Steele, 2006)

Although this chapter may seem irrelevant to the role of teachers, sadly there are a significant number of students in every school who are coping with such complex internal systems and they need to be treated with empathy and not frustration, until wholeness is possible where fragmentation currently exists.

HELPFUL RESPONSES TO A CHILD WHO IS DISSOCIATIVE

If you think a child could be dissociative, it is best to focus on being a consistent, predictable, reliable, empathetic, warm, kind and caring adult whilst also seeking to find professional help for them. These children need psychotherapy treatment from trauma specialists in order to facilitate a full recovery. When their behaviour is challenging, the key is to avoid shouting or unpredictable movements, as this can escalate the difficult behaviour. It is also important to avoid touching them in any way, including grabbing the child, unless absolutely necessary, and then to do so with clear, calm words of explanation and to allow time for processing afterwards. It is important to avoid labelling a child in any way and that the child sees that you care about them and want to help. Ultimately, a dissociative child is a highly courageous, intelligent child who has survived complex and tragic experiences that children should never be exposed to. Their recovery begins with stabilisation and safety, and a teacher can help to facilitate this by trying to create a classroom that is emotionally safe. Chapter 8 explores other strategies that facilitate making a classroom feel safer for children who are traumatised.

Discussion Points:

1. When a child has a 'full bucket' how does this affect their behaviour?

2. When a dissociative child is in the classroom, how do they act?

3. When a child is dissociative where do they fit on the trauma continuum?

4. Who needs to work with a dissociative child and why?

5. Do you think there is a dissociative child in your class and what will you now do to try and help them?

REDUCING STRESS
FOR TEACHERS
AND STUDENTS

CHAPTER 8

CLASSROOM STRATEGIES TO REDUCE STRESS

Research suggests that teachers are often aware of the centrality and importance of their role in the lives of traumatised children, yet they feel under-equipped to respond to the challenges of some confusing and volatile behaviour (de Thierry, 2014). Whilst they are often familiar with a wide range of trauma symptoms, they lack confidence in identifying appropriate strategies to support them. This is partially due to a lack of knowledge about trauma, but also to the pressure to focus on education standards. It is not being suggested that teachers should be encouraged to become mental health experts and to try to diagnose trauma, or even to treat those children who are affected differently, but instead to teach with an awareness that provides support and understanding for all children (Sitler, 2008). A speech therapist who trains professionals in trauma recovery, has expressed her similar desire to see all teachers have access to such information, in order to reduce stress for children and staff.

> 'One day, all teachers will be trained to detect possible trauma, all speech-language pathologists will be versed in the language of dissociation and all school psychologists will know to refer children for expert evaluation and help. One day schools will be a place for children to be truly safe.' (Wieland, 2010)

There are some key facts to remember when helping children, as the evidence suggests that having a teacher who understands the impact that trauma has on a child is already a positive strategy to facilitate a healthier, calmer, happier learning environment.

1. A psychological **trauma response to threat** causes a child's brain to act like an alarm, where the thinking, reasoning, analytical and negotiating ability of the brain goes 'off line' and the survival instinct takes over. When a child feels safe, then they are able to access their pre-frontal cortex and re-engage in thinking.

2. The broca area of the brain, which is responsible for speech and language, shuts down during trauma and **a child becomes 'speechless'.** This isn't a defiant response to annoy an adult and waste time, but a physiological response that they are unable to control. A child will often not be able to access words in order to describe a traumatic experience, even when they are calm and feel safe. It can take time to process the strong emotional response first before words can be used; hence creative therapy is a vital trauma intervention.

3. A child is often not aware that their negative behaviour is due to their traumatic experience and

they have **little cognitive ability to explain** what they are feeling and why they are behaving in that manner. Children are dependent upon a positive, engaging, warm relationship with an adult where they can learn how their body and emotions respond, and what they can do in response to this.

4. When a traumatised child has a positive experience at school, with at least one positive relationship that is predictable, nurturing, caring and warm, then they will be able to **form neural pathways** which can enable them to have positive relational experiences in the future.

5. As an adult we need to **model self-regulation** in order for children to learn this skill. A child will not learn how to manage strong emotions and negative experiences if they do not have an attachment figure who can help navigate them through these challenges and teach them the skills necessary.

6. Children's brains have a **high degree of plasticity** and are therefore able to change with relative ease compared to adults. This means that any investment into the lives of children and young people can replace the need for long-term support of a vulnerable adult.

7. Being an adult who is **warm, engaging, patient, and offers repetitive, rewarding, relational experiences** will eventually change the neural pathways of a traumatised child and enable them learn, relate to others and have dreams for their future.

8. **Shame increases negative behaviour** and any shame-inducing words or consequences need to be avoided at all cost.

OTHER STRATEGIES THAT CAN BE USED FOR CHILDREN WHO ARE SHOWING SIGNS OF TRAUMA

The first grouping is easy-to-remember approaches that help children to feel safe within a classroom.

PACE

Playful, Accepting, Curious and Empathetic (Hughes, 2009). This is a way to remember four essential attitudes to hold whilst relating to children. The main way that children process, think and work out life is through playing, and so to relate to a child through his or her natural language is the easiest way to engage and understand them. To be accepting, curious and empathetic are important relational approaches that demonstrate that a child has value and an adult's role is not just to tell a child what to do, but to listen, learn, accept and be interested in a child's world. Ultimately, this is showing respect to a child as a person who has a right to their own feelings, thoughts and perspectives.

CARES

Communicate Alternatively, Release Endorphins, Self-Soothe (Ferenz, 2012). CARES is a specifically designed way to help a child or young person to self-regulate when they are in distress. Ferenz writes that it is a model to:

> 'Help clients achieve, in healthier ways, the same positive gains they get from self-destructive

*behaviours. Most clients are tuned in to the fact
that self-destructive behaviours ameliorate tension
and anxiety, and quell the re-surfacing of painful
memories and affect.'*

It is a quick way to help a child feel that their feelings
are validated yet seeks a way to communicate them in a
manner that helps them to enable everyone to stay safe.
For example, a child who is kicking another child can
be taken aside and reminded that whilst it is noted that
they may feel frustrated, would they like to thump the
angry cushion instead. A child is taught to understand
their own trauma responses and know that they need
to find an alternative way to communicate their feelings
rather than deny that they exist. They are then taught
that to counteract the cortisol flooding through their
body they can choose to undertake activities that release
endorphins, such as running around a playground three
times, performing star jumps in the corridor, or using
a punch-bag. This is then followed by a self-soothing
activity that validates the difficulty encountered by these
strong reactions and feelings, such as listening to music,
snuggling under a blanket with a soft toy, or reading a
story.

PATIENCE AND WARMTH

A traumatised child is highly attuned and hypervigilant
in order to be ready for threat or disaster. This means that
they will possibly notice what mood adults are in, even
before they may have noticed themselves! It is preferable
that a teacher is always calm, patient, warm and gentle
with children, but when this goes wrong then they can

use it as an opportunity to model reflection, by using sentences such as: *'Oh dear, I do think I feel a bit grumpy today. I am sorry. Now let me take a few minutes to reflect on why, so that I can be a cheerful teacher.'* This would calm frightened children and empower them to respond to their own feelings in such a manner.

When a child picks up the feeling that a teacher is frustrated with them, it can cause a child who was feeling just slightly on edge to explode due to overwhelming feelings of fear, guilt or failure. Sometimes as adults we like to think that we can say something positive and squeeze out a smile, but a hypervigilant child picks up on the feelings inside us by watching every muscle on our face move and can read between the words that we speak.

Patience and warmth speak volumes to a child who has been under-nurtured, and can heal a traumatised child so that they feel they can begin to take risks to learn or try something new. Patience can never be underestimated as a vital strategy to support the troubled child. When things get busy and challenging, patience can still be found by utilising the skill of empathy; 'standing in their shoes' and picturing the internal pain that they are in.

AVOIDING SHAME AT ALL COST

It is acknowledged that many discipline approaches adopt shame inadvertently as a way of punishing children and encouraging them to improve their behaviour. We, however, believe that children who have been traumatised often have a history of shame due to their traumatic experiences, and so further shame escalates negative behaviour. We work hard to motivate a child to be in control of their behaviour because they appreciate the feeling of being good and are relieved to behave in a way that is expected. We avoid all shame in any situation, as there is nothing of value in the experience of shame.

WORDS THAT FACILITATE A CALM ATMOSPHERE

The way that we speak can either create a calm environment or cause children to feel anxious or be easily triggered. Whilst the most foundational way to speak to a traumatised child is through warmth and kindness, there are other skills regarding words that enable a child to feel listened to rather than controlled. When a child feels controlled, they are very much more likely to respond from a threat or alarm state.

Unhelpful words	Helpful words
Please be quiet and just tell me what's wrong	I am wondering if you feel frustrated right now and you want me to listen to you?
Stop whining like a baby	I think you've got something important to say. Take a deep breath and then I can listen to you.
No one is going to listen to you when you make such an awful noise. Grow up.	I think you're struggling to use words at the moment, so maybe I can help you. Shall we breathe together and then get your special teddy?

The second grouping is a few general strategies that can help calm a frightened child:

GROUNDING

This is a term which describes helping someone who is frightened to remember that they can stay in the 'here and now' and calm themselves. The first part of grounding someone is to use a calming tone of voice that gently speaks to a child and tells them that you are there to support them. They can then be informed of where they are and what has just happened if they exhibit signs of confusion. The second part of grounding is to help a child breathe in a way that calms them down, by taking some big, long, slow breaths in and out and to feel these breaths. The third step is to help a child understand these cognitive calming words. When they are in a state of terror, the best way to do this is through the use of sensory stimuli, such as strong smells, or textured toys to fiddle with, or anything that moves all the neural energy from the brainstem. You could try music or comforting smelling hand-cream, or you could suggest that they eat chewing gum to stimulate their taste buds and release endorphins through the chewing action. When they are feeling safe and soothed, but may be feeling a sense of shame or confusion, you can stimulate their cortex by asking them to tell you a joke or a tongue twister. Help them to feel their feet on the ground and to feel their rhythmical breathing. Stay with them until they are calm and can speak to you, and avoid any fast, aggressive, threatening, judging or angry words or behaviours.

REASSURING

Let a child know that they are safe and use the tone of your voice to reassure them through a gentle, non-judgemental, warm and understanding approach. This approach will speed up the process of a child becoming calm, because they feel safer. When a child feels judged, mocked or misunderstood, then their negative behaviour escalates. A child needs to view the adult as responsible and in control so that they don't have to stay in a hyperalert and hypervigilant state in case of further danger. It can sometimes be important to explain what has just happened, if a child feels confused or dissociated during the escalation. For example, it can be helpful to explain calmly that they just ran out of the room screaming, which was probably because there was a big loud noise because a chair was pushed over by mistake. A child can then be reassured that no one is angry with them and it's all going to be OK. Allow them to ask questions about the incident, as this helps a child to feel safe and become calm, and enables them to become calmer faster during subsequent occasions.

UNDERSTANDING

Explaining to a child that you understand that they feel scared, angry or frustrated and helping them to understand that these feelings are validated is helpful. When they feel less frightened about your response, you can gently ask them to take some big, deep breaths which will help children de-escalate and be able to think (see calm breathing guide). Understanding that a child can find it difficult to access their thinking brain or words can increase our patience as adults as we focus instead on breathing and calming a child. It is also time-efficient to make an effort to ask other professionals who are working with a child to see if they have discovered what triggers cause a trauma response, so that these can be avoided if possible.

HELPING CHILDREN TO SELF-SOOTHE

A child needs to have their strong feelings and responses validated, not so that they increase, rather so that they can be reduced. A child also needs to have worked out what is soothing for them when they are recovering from an incident, such as a special cuddly toy, a writing journal or a blanket with a special smell that is comforting.

CALMING BREATHING TECHNIQUE

This can be used when a child has become distressed to calm them and is something that they will then learn to do themselves.

> Take a slow breath in through the nose (for about 4 seconds)
> Hold your breath for 1 or 2 seconds
> Exhale slowly through the mouth (over about 4 seconds)
> Wait 2-3 seconds before taking another breath (5-7 seconds for teenagers)
> Repeat for at least 5 to 10 breaths

SPECIFIC STRATEGIES FOR THE CLASSROOM

This third grouping presents some specific strategies that can be useful for a child but are dependent on each individual child and their unique needs and fears.

FOR CHILDREN WHO ARE ON THE LOWER END OF THE TRAUMA CONTINUUM AND ARE SHOWING SIGNS OF STRESS

- They could use a laminated sheet of emotion faces all day to show how they feel.
- When a child has attachment issues, they need a key person whom they can tell if they are worried; this person can facilitate them being able to check in after transitions or changes.
- It can also be essential to reflect on the seating positions within a classroom and to ensure that there is an easy escape route and a good place to run to.
- Positive, specific affirmation can be reassuring that a child has been noticed and valued.
- A child can be given roles and responsibilities that they can perform to increase their confidence.
- They could also be given roles that facilitate physical activity to help them regulate, for example, take the register, look for a 'missing' toy.
- Most children find a visual timetable helpful for predictability.
- Sometimes stress balls and fiddly toys can be subtly used for calming.
- Some children find doodle books and mosaic

colouring books helpful for self-soothing.

- Use reflection diaries and sheets to develop the skill of reflection and begin to develop the skill of recognising and beginning to understand the impact of behaviour on others.
- There can be a tactile area in the classroom with beanbags, rocking chairs or plush rugs that offer children support to calm down whilst also enabling them to stay with the class.
- Activities can be facilitated that promote the child's sense of strengths and interests.
- Make a calm down bottle with each child in the class. Find a bottle that can be squeezed, fill a quarter full of glitter glue, top with warm water and a few objects such as lego men. Seal the top! The child then squeezes the bottle when they feel agitated or angry and can watch the glitter and wait for the lego man to appear.

FOR CHILDREN WHO ARE IN THE MIDDLE OF THE TRAUMA CONTINUUM

- Ensure that information on trauma is available for all those working with the child.
- Go out to the playground if possible to observe behaviour and dynamics.
- Don't feel bad about making allowances for children who need individual strategies.
- Provide a struggling child with an emergency sign 'red' traffic light which they can display in order to ask to leave the classroom due to panic or frustration.
- Use a marble jar and ask children to pop a marble in each time they feel stressed during the day. This can be

helpful to show escalation.
- Facilitate sensory time if it is appropriate to de-escalate and ground a child.
- Enable the child to have somewhere safe to run to if they need to run.
- Pair up an older pupil who is a mentor to help a traumatised child during playtimes.
- Facilitate stretching, short burst exercises or relaxation activities into the day's programme at regular times.
- Have a calm box with things that the child needs to help them self regulate, such as their chosen toy, special photos and sensory items.
- Make sure that instructions are short, clear and repeated often to help the students whose memory is being challenged due to extreme stress.
- Use clocks in different positions in the room and verbalise the length of each session and how long remains to help the child grasp a sense of time.
- Make sure that the class code of conduct and any behaviour expectations are clearly reinforced using a range of methods.
- Make sure that the child can 'check in' each day and each week with how they are finding school and how they are feeling about friends and family.
- Providing a structure for some play times with group games or sports equipment for use on their own.
- Provide music in the classroom to calm the children.
- Understand that events like assembly where large groups are gathered in quiet can cause high levels of anxiety, which can lead to negative behaviour caused by the threat response.

FOR CHILDREN ON THE COMPLEX TRAUMA END OF THE CONTINUUM

For children who are dissociative and on the furthest end of the trauma continuum: these children, on the top corner of the trauma triangle, need a bespoke strategy that is written according to their specific internal system and specific triggers and needs and parts. An approach needs to be worked through with the whole team around the child. The lead should be taken from the complex trauma expert, who can advise on the treatment plan and expectations of the recovery journey.

Again, it is important to note that the standard assessment tool that is used with children, the SDQ (strengths and difficulties questionaire), *does not* identify complex trauma; therefore it can be common for the most traumatised children to miss out on therapeutic interventions as their SDQ score could present as lower than a child on the lower end of the trauma contiuum. It is also vital to note that the highly traumatised child's brain will not have the cognitive functioning capacity to process verbal and cognitive therapy approaches. They need creative therapies that are not dependant on verbal processing, in order to access the right brain implicit memory.

Children who have complex trauma must be referred to trauma specialists as the strategies need to be tailored for each specific case. They need small class sizes with therapeutic support workers.

THE GROUP DYNAMIC

While these approaches may seem time-consuming and add to the complexity of the role, they need not take much time, and they can de-escalate, rather than escalate, a problem and so ultimately should save you time.

You may be concerned that other children in the class will resent the 'special treatment' that one child is receiving. However (and especially if a child is aggressive or explosive), other pupils often welcome fewer dramatic incidents. Other students often end up also following the teacher's modelling of offering support and compassion if a child gets upset.

Discussion Points:

1. What fact have you learned about trauma that will have the most impact upon your classroom practice?

2. What approach do you find the easiest?

3. What approach do you find the hardest?

4. What general strategies do you feel confident to use?

5. What strategies are you going to try in the coming weeks?

CHAPTER 9

ATTACHMENT TO
A TEACHER

In the first decade of a child's life, a classroom teacher is a primary attachment figure because of the amount of time spent together within the classroom setting. Of course, this relational need becomes challenging to a teacher if a child has no other consistent attachment figures and there are 30 other children sharing the one teacher. This can of course add to the stress and exhaustion that teachers can feel, but it can also motivate them further to try and identify who is in need of the attachment experience the most, and how they can facilitate a feeling of being safe within the classroom. In the secondary classroom, amidst many different teachers who teach hundreds of children each day, it can be easy to avoid all attachment to any adults, but after speaking to young people for many years, I have found that they knew which teachers seemed to care, understand and show empathy. Teachers can make the difference by just taking notice of the lives of the traumatised children in their classes.

When a child is traumatised through unpredictable relationships, they can become untrusting of the external world to keep them safe. They then distrust their own feelings because they are not acknowledged and verbalised and they can stop seeking comfort. It is easier for them to keep everyone at a safe distance away and disconnect. Teachers can however, become an adult that they recognize as predictable and protective and this can facilitate healing.

Marcus and Sanders-Reio (2001) found that attachment to teachers affected educational motivation. They discovered that when a teacher was attuned, caring and consistent, the student was more able to learn because they felt safer and calmer. Children with attachment disruptions or insecure attachments found classrooms difficult, due to the intense social and emotional dynamics, which are often areas that can be full of anxiety when trust is not a norm. Research has shown (de Thierry, 2014) that when teachers understand this factor, attitudes within classrooms change as they found that they were naturally more attuned and empathetic to the students, and were aware of the need for repetitive, relational, consistent, and predictable experiences. When I was interviewing teachers undertaking the 'Understanding Trauma' course that I run for teachers, consistent comments were made, such as:

> 'The main thing I have learnt from the Understanding Trauma course, is to watch pupils more closely and be aware of their reaction to situations, myself, other staff, pupils, surroundings and lesson content – to build up a picture about them – not to jump to conclusions, understand that they are traumatised, and to have an awareness of them as people going through more than just your particular lesson. I now try and put myself in their shoes.' (Claire)

Teachers could feel overwhelmed by filling all the roles of one who educates, identifies, refers, supports, listens to, helps, models healthy attachment, and facilitates recovery within the context of a healthy, understanding, empathetic relationship. However, our research indicates that these roles seemed natural and became less draining when a teacher felt confident as a result of understanding the neuroscience of trauma, the symptoms of trauma, and some easy intervention strategies. There is no suggestion that this knowledge is the only answer to relieving the stress associated with the teacher's role, but it did provide significant reassurance and stress relief regarding challenging children who had previously caused them confusion. The research evidenced that there was a reduction in anxiety following a trauma training course that included knowledge found in this book. The Likert-type scale used in the research revealed that there was a transformation from 90% of the teachers attending feeling anxious about the well-being of some young people in the classroom and what to do about it, to only 10% feeling anxious (de Thierry, 2014).

The mental health professionals Geary (2007), Allisic (2012), Howard (2013), Sitler (2008), Greenhalgh (1994) and others, all concur that the role of teachers has the possibility to facilitate the recovery of traumatised children. Research suggests that the teacher-student relationship can be a source of recovery from traumatic experiences, and some would assert that this relationship may be the most important factor for positive adaptation to school, in providing role models and emotional support (Alisic et al., 2012).

A teacher's relationship with a traumatised child can result in enhanced neurological function, and improved behavioural and overall well-being outcomes for children, due to the close, caring and supportive role of a teacher (Howard, 2013). This is achievable if teachers are equipped with an understanding of attachment theory and the impact of trauma upon a child, because they then tend not to question whether it was something that they did that created a child's negative response, and instead they understand that 'these outbursts are very likely for a child of trauma, even in the most supportive of environments.' (Howard, 2013).

RELATIONSHIPS THAT ENABLE A CHILD TO RECOVER FROM TRAUMA ARE:

The adult offers repeated, rewarding relational interactions.

The adult is warm, empathetic engaging, curious and kind.

The adult is consistent and predictable in their communication.

The adult validates the child's feelings.

The child experiences an adult protecting them.

The child experiences an adult trying to take care of them.

A TRAUMATISED CHILD'S NEED FOR POSITIVE ADULT RELATIONSHIPS

Perry (2011) presents the argument that some traumatised children have so few positive relational experiences that they are not able to develop the capacity to be socially appropriate, empathetic and self-regulating. He suggests that, often, by the time they reach ten, they have only had the number and quality of positive relational social experiences that a typical five-year-old has experienced. Teachers can facilitate a positive relational experience, which can change the expectations of children who have not had the benefit of enjoying an adult's care and nurture. This doesn't need to take additional time but just the recognition that every smile, every look of affirmation, every validation of a feeling, and every time comfort is offered, can change the neurological pathways of a child's brain forever, and thereby change their future.

As one teacher wrote with wisdom after their first year of work:

> 'At the end of my first year of teaching, I am left with one thin, elusive but crucial strand of idealism: if I can make a difference in one child's life, if one child finds some self-worth in my class, if one child makes something of themselves, then I have done my job. I am a teacher.' (Rogers, 2004)

Understanding the impact of trauma on a child helps teachers to relate to their students in a helpful, healing, consistent, and emotionally regulating way, whilst also continuing to primarily be an educator.

Discussion Points:

1. What small approaches can you adopt which can radically change the life of a traumatised child?

2. Can you remember the name of a teacher from your childhood who was influential in your life?

3. As a teacher who works with traumatised children each day, what can you do to make sure that you are emotionally supported?

4. How can a teacher adopt time for reflection during the busy nature of a school day?

CHAPTER 10

SECONDARY TRAUMA AND TEACHERS' STRESS

Research has shown that teachers develop more positive emotional responses to children almost immediately after learning about the impact of trauma on a child (de Thierry, 2014). Teachers reported that they felt less impatient, irritable and frustrated, and felt an increase in calm and confidence. One of the reasons for this reduction in negative emotion is the understanding that a child may be responding to trauma, and as a result, the child's anger, defiance and unpleasant behaviour no longer have such a personal effect on the teacher. Teachers articulated that, after learning about trauma, they were relieved to have a clear cognitive ability to de-personalise the verbal attacks and rejection of children in the classroom. They found immediate consolation when they learned that the responses of these children were caused by outside influences and were able to offer support, rather than feel defensive. This came from an understanding of the definitions and experiences of transference and projection, concepts that are familiar to a psychotherapist yet not commonly explained to teachers, who are often at the receiving end of such complex psychological interactions. The following is a quotation from an experienced teacher who learnt the definitions of these terms whilst attending the training course and subsequently noticed a reduction in her feelings of failure and powerlessness:

> *'I have been less reactive to behaviour and more able to respond in a calm manner, separating my personal anxiety and realising it is them who is feeling anxious. I focus on the individual and form a relationship that is suited to their needs; in a professional manner of course.'* (Julia)

This was echoed by other teachers in another study and has also been a common response in school settings in other nations where such information is distributed to schools:

> *'We often find that adults who have an understanding of attachment theory and the impact of trauma to students tend to fare better. They tend not to question whether it was something they did (or did not do) that led to the event. Rather they acknowledge that these outbursts are very likely for a child of trauma, even in the most supportive of environments.'* (Howard, 2013)

When a teacher understands that a traumatised child has a psychological need to control a situation due to constant feelings of fear and vulnerability, they are more able to manage their own reactions. A teacher is then enabled to manage their own feelings of powerlessness and frustration when they understand that the child is primarily dealing with strong feelings of fear, rather than wanting to be rebellious.

SECONDARY TRAUMA

Teacher stress is a subject that has been articulated in the media due to increasing pressure on outcomes, including the introduction of OFSTED, league tables, and other such public methods of critiquing the profession. What is rarely acknowledged is the possibility of secondary trauma for teachers who are providing support to the escalating numbers of children and young people who are struggling emotionally. Secondary trauma occurs when the emotions that have been projected onto a caring adult begin to affect them without the ability to manage them; this is conceivably due to a lack of time to reflect on and process these feelings.

O'Hara (2014) highlighted the problem of teachers having to 'pick up the pieces from cuts to youth mental health services', and a head teacher that she interviewed for her article in The Guardian newspaper raised the issue that 'teachers are not mental health professionals.' This professional pressure, alongside the knowledge of secondary trauma, is worrying, yet educating teachers about the symptoms of vicarious trauma can start to equip them to deal appropriately with early signs, and thereby avoid long-term health problems.

"When working with disturbed children, one might find oneself feeling hurt, abused, angry, frustrated, intolerant, anxious, de-skilled and even frightened."
(Greenhalgh, 1994, p.53)

Psychological research has provided evidence of the power of another person's empathy to build resilience in order to help with stressful experiences (Cozolino, 2006; Perry, 2011). Research suggests that teachers who work with traumatised children should not only be equipped with an understanding of secondary trauma, but should also be provided with appropriate emotional support and empathy from a supervisor or line manager. This emotional provision would enhance teachers' classroom practice, benefit their well-being, and avoid emotional burnout by facilitating the avoidance of secondary trauma.

REFLECTIVE TIME, SELF-AWARENESS, SELF-REGULATION AND SUPPORT

The need for reflection time and the opportunity to talk with peers about the expressions of trauma that occur in classrooms seems to be a crucial factor for teachers' well-being. In the literature exploring teachers' roles and perceptions of their relationships with and influences on the children they teach (Sitler, 2008), a repeated theme emerges concerning their need to be equipped with methods of helping them.

Trauma is an experience that isolates children and causes internal shattering, and teachers who are involved in the daily care of traumatised children can experience similar internal, emotional responses to the resulting classroom behaviour (Howard, 2013). Half of the teachers who participated in a study of the experience of supporting traumatised children indicated a difficulty with emotional involvement (Alisic et al., 2012). For other emotionally involved professionals, the risk of compassion fatigue is recognised and support strategies are offered, but there is currently no acknowledgment of such a need for teachers, even though they are more involved and interact daily with traumatised children. Counsellors and psychotherapists have to complete a number of hours of clinical supervision in order to meet the regulation requirements (British Association for Counselling & Psychotherapy; BACP; 2013) and to ensure that they have adequate space to reflect on the intense work of supporting those affected by trauma. In contrast, teachers are often left without time to reflect, emotional support or an understanding of the nature and relational consequences of trauma for children and for others involved in those children's lives. Ellis (2012) writes of the importance of those working with traumatised people having space to process thoughts about their observations and their own emotional responses to them.

Pritzker (2012) also asserts that there is a need for reflective practice. He has studied teachers' responses to students' unsettling behaviour in schools, and argues that for teachers (as indeed for all individuals), painful school memories offer an important source of information on identity construction. Such memories form foundational beliefs in the subconscious mind of a teacher, which could affect their emotional response to their work. He argues that while most education professionals have neglected to facilitate a discussion around emotion responses for many years, education and teaching research has recently focused upon emotions as a component of teacher identity, suggesting that they act as a lens through which identity can be investigated. Pritzker has explored unresolved early childhood memories and repressed pain, which can lead to hesitant and restrained behaviour patterns within the classroom. He concludes that both novice and experienced teachers should examine and reflect upon their negative life experiences and support should be provided to process them in a safe and non-judging setting.

In order to be a safe, warm, empathetic adult in a traumatised child's life, it is essential to model self-regulation skills and help the child to see them work. To be an emotionally regulated adult enables a traumatised child to be less defensive, fearful and expecting of danger. When their hypervigilance is reduced because they can see that their teacher is able to keep them safe, then they are able to access their learning brain and can also begin to build attachments with others, as they are less defensive and ready for danger. In order for teachers to stay self-regulated in the face of a stressful, demanding job, it seems that a supportive team, self-awareness, reflective thinking and either supervision or line management that includes care for the individual person, rather than just the work achieved, are essential.

Ultimately, it seems that teachers are often left with a demanding, important and fulfilling role that sometimes has insufficient emotional support because of the rise in the number of traumatised children who are sitting in the classrooms of today. However, it does seem that if a teacher is able to be emotionally self-regulated, can offer care and genuine warmth to the children they teach and has an understanding of the impact of trauma, then they can be the most influential people in the lives of these vulnerable young individuals with the power to change the path of their future.

We need to facilitate a change in culture today so that teachers are valued as the influencers of today and tomorrow, and are also given the necessary support to enjoy and flourish in their role, rather than to leave the profession exhausted and discouraged because of the few who were unable to respond well.

I shall end with the words of two pioneers in trauma recovery, and it is encouraging to remember that recovery is possible for many through the use of the simplest of methods.

> 'Fortunately, however, there is an antidote even to uncomfortable stress, one that is not necessarily out of reach for even the poorest of the poor. And that of course is the kindness of others, the nurturing contact that is designed to put the brakes on the chemistry of fear and threat. When children are raised by stressed parents in chronically stressful circumstances, the stress engine can become more powerful and the brakes weaker and less able to slow it down. Nonetheless, the patterned, repetitive experience can build it up.' (Perry and Szalavitz, 2010)

APPENDIX A

THE TRC'S OAKSIDE CREATIVE EDUCATIONAL CENTRE CORE VALUES

Oakside Creative Education Centre is a project of the TRC. It is an alternative education provision for children and young people who are too traumatised to engage in mainstream education. Most children have experienced multiple exclusions.

At Oakside Creative Education Centre we have certain expectations about a child's journey with us, including what that will look like and our key objectives along the way. This central values document introduces the key concepts that are often different to mainstream primary or secondary schools.

VIOLENT OR AGGRESSIVE BEHAVIOUR

Here at Oakside we adamantly believe that children do not want to be bad or be told off. We believe that all children desire to be praised and admired. Therefore we believe that when a child is caught in a cycle of destructive behaviour it is for various reasons, and it's our job as the adults to try and work out why. We spend a lot of time observing children's reactions to different experiences in order to ascertain what could cause them to behave in unhelpful ways. We 'map' each child's individual triggers, frustrations, fears and struggles so that we can break the cycle of negative behaviour.

When they are violent or aggressive we adamantly believe that they feel the need to protect themselves and we want to find out why. We believe that fear is the primary reason for aggression, unless it is a learnt behaviour from what they have viewed on screens or from personal experience. As staff we are trained in the Team Teach approach of de-escalation, with restraint as the last option. We would hope that as we journey together the restraining incidents would drop to zero within a short time frame of us mapping their behaviour and teaching them new method's to cope with difficult feelings. We believe that their behaviour is almost always the children trying to speak to us without words and so we try and understand what they are trying to tell us.

We are also aware that the children themselves usually feel embarrassed or ashamed of any violent or aggressive behaviour, and usually feel that they have to deal with negative emotions by 'acting hard' or pretending not to care. We do not 'tell them off' but wait until they have calmed down and feel safe, before discussing with them what has happened.

DAYDREAMING OR A LACK OF FOCUS

Often children who have been traumatised are told off for daydreaming or being unable to focus on their work. We adamantly believe that this is because the children are using all their energy to survive, and thus the primary place of neural activity is in the brainstem. The brainstem is the reptilian part of the brain which is responsible for the fright, flight and freeze response, and is highly active when a child feels under threat. This preoccupation with survival doesn't allow a child to easily access the other parts of brain, which allow for negotiation, reasoning or analysing. Therefore, we know that often a child will be in the freeze response and not be able to hear what a teacher says or to respond appropriately. Daydreaming can feel like the safest place for a child whilst they are unsafe in their circumstances. This trauma symptom dramatically reduces as a child recovers due to appropriate trauma therapy.

CHANGES IN PERSONALITY

We recognise that children often have rapid behaviour changes, such as being calm and easy going, and then suddenly becoming angry and unreasonable, before switching to frightened and timid. We recognise that trauma can cause a child to adopt coping mechanisms which can trigger sudden, and sometimes shocking and conflicting, responses which seem to 'come from nowhere'. We believe that these are coping mechanisms and so we expect to work with a child in order to understand what has happened as part of our 'mapping'. These behaviour changes begin to be less marked as children feel safer and therapy facilitates their recovery.

AVOIDING SHAME AT ALL COST

We recognise that many discipline approaches adopt shame inadvertently as a way of punishing children and encouraging them to improve their behaviour. However, we believe that children who have been traumatised often have a history of shame due to their traumatic experiences and so further shame escalates negative behaviour. We work hard to motivate a child to be in control of their behaviour because they appreciate the feeling of being good and are relieved to behave in a way that is expected. We avoid all shame in any situation, as there is nothing of value in the experience of shame.

LYING AND MAKING UP STORIES

We recognise that many children use lies and made-up stories to protect themselves from the reality of their own life experience. We understand this and do not feel the need to challenge them unless there is a specific need for truth. Lying can be a trauma symptom, and as such we would expect there to be a reduction of it during their time with us.

THE POWER OF EMPATHY

Neuroscience has revealed what the therapeutic world already knew, that empathy can create an environment where healing can take place. As the adults at Oakside, we adopt an empathetic approach; we try and see the world from our students' eyes and respond from that place. We believe that as we respond with compassion and warmth, a child develops an ability to respect themselves and care for themselves. Empathy is vital to demonstrate an interest in a child and form a positive attachment.

TEACHING SELF-REGULATION

At Oakside we place a high value on teaching children the skills of self-regulation. This involves the skill of somatic recognition and thus each day time is spent helping children recognise the feelings in their body. This enables them to develop ways to respond to triggers as they begin to recognise the very beginning of their escalating response. The children learn to recognise feelings in their heads, tummies, hands and legs, and they learn how to respond and then how to utilise the sofa and story time, the tent, the water and sensory activities, and drums. The children develop the skill of recognising emotions and regulating their responses. We expect that the children who come to us to exhibit unregulated behaviour and to return to full time mainstream school able to self-regulate their emotions, responses and reactions.

THE IMPORTANCE OF PLAY

We believe that play is not an optional extra for children, as we believe that children process their challenges and work out life through their play. Consequently, we facilitate children to play as a vital part of their welfare and recovery. Children need free play to process what's on their mind and they need directive play to help them navigate challenges and learn social skills. At Oakside, play is timetabled more than in mainstream schools so that their recovery can be faster.

THE IMPORTANCE OF SENSORY WORK

Sensory work is built into the timetable at Oakside because we recognise the neurobiological benefits for children. Research has shown that trauma and sensory deprivation in the child-parent relationship may be an underlying cause of a number of emotional disturbances in children, including anxiety, depression, attention deficit, aggression and attachment disorders, and sensory integration dysfunction (Prescott, 1971; Van Der Kolk, 1996;, Kranowitz, 1998). During sensory play activities neural connectors are increased and trauma induced brain damage can be repaired (Perry, 2004; Siegel, 2004).

THE IMPORTANCE OF ATTACHMENT

We recognise the value of attachment, and consequently we ensure consistency in our staff team. We know that children flourish when they experience repetitive, rewarding and relationally rich experiences. We adopt the Hughes method of PACE and work in a playful, accepting, curious and empathetic manner with the children. We know that these children need the staff to help them develop positive relational experiences that enable them to recover.

> "Some children have so few positive relational experiences that they don't develop the capacity to be socially appropriate, empathic, self-regulating and humane. By the time they reach age 10, they have only had the number and quality of positive social interactions that a typical 5 year old gets."
> (Perry 2006)

BETSY DE THIERRY, 2014

This document can be copied and used to aid schools' understanding, if credit is given to the TRC, Oakside and the author.

APPENDIX B

ORGANISATIONS THAT OFFER EXPERTISE IN TRAUMA OR COMPLEX TRAUMA

The Trauma Recovery Centre (TRC) offers training and consultations for schools, and therapy for traumatised children and young people. *www.trc-uk.org*

The Institute of Recovery from Childhood Trauma (IRCT) is an umbrella organisation that exists to ensure that recovery from childhood trauma is available for all. *www.irct.uk.org*

The European Study of Trauma and Dissociation (ESTD) www.estd.org and the International Society for the Study of Trauma and Dissociation (ISSTD) offer expertise on complex trauma and has a fact sheet for teachers to download. *www.isst-d.org*

The Child Trauma Academy offers expertise on

trauma and the impact on children through courses, books and newsletters. *www.childtrauma.org*

The National Child Traumatic Stress Network also has great resources for teachers and parents about trauma and supporting the traumatised child. *www.nctsn.org*

LOOKING FOR A THERAPIST?

Looking for a therapist for a child? Here are some national organisations to help find a therapist (below websites accessed in January 2015).

British Association of Counsellors and Psychotherapists: http://www.bacpregister.org.uk

UK Council for Psychotherapists:
http://members.psychotherapy.org.uk/findATherapist

Gestalt London:
http://gestaltcentre.co.uk/what-is-gestalt/

British Association of Music Therapists:
http://www.bamt.org

British Association of Art Therapists:
http://www.baat.org

Play Therapists UK:
http://www.playtherapyregister.org.uk

British Association of Play Therapists:
http://www.bapt.info/find-therapist/

HELPFUL CORE BOOKS FOR THE FURTHER EXPLORATION OF TRAUMA

FOR TEACHERS TO DEVELOP FURTHER UNDERSTANDING

Cozolino, L. (2006)
The Neuroscience of Human Relationships. Attachment and the Social Brain
New York: Norton Publishers

Perry, B. & Szalavitz, M. (2011).
Born for Love: Why Empathy Is Essential and Endangered
New York: Harper Collins

Siegel. D. Bryson. T. (2012).
The Whole Brain Child. Revolutionary strategies to nurture your child's developing mind
Robinson Publishing

FOR CLINICIANS AND PROFESSIONALS WHO WORK 1:1 TO UNDERSTAND TRAUMA TREATMENT

Levine. P. & Kline. M. (2006)
Trauma through a child's eyes
California. North Atlantic Books

FOR CLINICIANS TO UNDERSTAND COMPLEX TRAUMA

Wieland, S. (2010)
Dissociation in Traumatised Children and Adolescents
New York. Routledge

REFERENCES

Alisic, E. (2012)
Teachers' perspectives on providing support to children after trauma: a qualitative study
School Psychology Quarterly, 27(1), 51-59

Allen, J.G. (2003)
Mentalizing
Bulletin of the Menninger Clinic, 67(2), 212-226

American Psychiatric Publishing (2013)
Diagnostic and statistical manual of mental disorders, Fifth edition (DSM-5)
Washington, DC: American Psychiatric Publishing

British Association for Counselling and Psychotherapy, BACP (2013)
Ethical framework for good practice in counselling and psychotherapy
British Association for Counselling and Psychotherapy
Available from: http://www.bacp.co.uk /ethical_framework/ (Accessed 23/10/13)

Baginsky, M. (2003)
Newly qualified teachers and child protection
Child Abuse Review, 12, 119-127

BBC News UK Online (2013)
One in ten young people cannot cope with 'daily life', 2nd Jan 2013
Available from: http://www.bbc.co.uk/news/uk-20885838. (Accessed 18/03/13)

Beaulieu, D. (2003)
Eye Movement Integration Therapy: the comprehensive clinical guide
Carmarthen: Crown House Publishing

Bowlby, J. (1998)
A secure base
London and New York: Routledge

Children and Family Court Advisory and Support Service, Cafcass (2009)
Care statistics continue to rise
Press release 8th May 2009. London: Cafcass
Available from: http://www.cafcass.gov.uk/news/archive/2009/care-statistics.aspx. (Accessed 12/06/13)

Cozolino, L. (2006).
The neuroscience of human relationships. Attachment and the social brain
New York: Norton Publishers

Daniel, M. (2014).
Tackling mental illness. Children and Young People Now
18th February-3rd March 2014

Department for Education, (2011)
Support and aspiration: a new approach to special educational needs and disability: a consultation
Department for Education, London: The Stationery Office
Available from: (https://www.gov.uk/government/ publications/ support-and-aspiration-a-new-approach-to-special-educational-needs-and-disability-consultation. Accessed 12/12/13)

Donnelly, L. (2013)
Children as young as five suffering from depression
The Daily Telegraph. 30th September 2013
Available from: http://www.telegraph.co.uk/ health/ healthnews/10342447/Children-as-young-as-five-suffering-from-depression. html (Accessed 21/10/13).

Downey, L. (2009). From isolation to connection
A guide to understanding and working with traumatised children and young people
Melbourne: Office of the Child Safety Commissioner
Available from: http://www.ccyp.vic.gov.au/ childsafetycommissioner/
downloads/isolation-to-connection-september-2009.pdf (Accessed:
02/02/14)

Ellis, G. (2012)
The impact on teachers of supporting children exposed to domestic violence
Educational and Child Psychology, 29(4)

Ferentz, L. (2012)
Treating self- destructive behaviors in trauma survivors. Working with the cycle: self-destructive behaviors and CARESS
New York: Routledge Press.

Geary, B. (2007)
Calmer Classrooms. A guide to working with traumatised children
Melbourne: Office of the Child Safety Commissioner
State Government Victoria
Available from: http://www.ccyp.vic.gov.au/search-results.
htm?q=safer+ classrooms& as_sitesearch=http%3A%2F%2Fwww.
ccyp.vic.gov.au&btnG=search. (Accessed 08/05/13).

Ginott, H.G. (1975)
Teacher and child: a book for parents and teachers
New York: Macmillan

Greenhalgh, P. (1994)
Emotional growth and learning
New York: Routledge

Heide, K. & Solomon, E. (1999)
Type III trauma: toward a more effective conceptualization of psychological trauma
International Journal of Offender Therapy and Comparative
Criminology, 43(2), 202-210

Howard, J.A. (2012)
Distressed or deliberately defiant?
Queensland, Australia: Australian Academic Press Group Pty. Ltd.

Hughes, D. (2009)
Attachment focused parenting
New York: Norton

ISSTD (2009)
Child and Adolescent Committee (2009): Frequently asked questions for teachers
The International Society for the Study of Trauma and Dissociation
Available at: http://www.isst-d.org/education/faq-teachers.htm.

James, B. (1989)
Treating traumatised children
Glencoe, IL: The Free Press

Kenny, M. (2004)
Teachers' attitudes toward and knowledge of child maltreatment
Child Abuse and Neglect, 28, 1311-1319

Marcus, R.F. & Sanders-Reio, J. (2001)
The influence of attachment on school completion
School Psychology Quarterly, 16(4), 427-444

McKee, B.E. & Dillenburger, K. (2009)
Child abuse and Neglect: training needs of student teachers
International Journal of Educational Research 48, 320-330

National Child Traumatic Stress Network (2008)
Child trauma toolkit for educators
Available from: www.nctsn.org/ nctsn _assets/PDFs/Child_Trauma_
Toolkit_Final.pdf (Accessed 12/4/12)

OFSTED (2013)
School-led partnerships setting the benchmark for high quality teacher training
Press release 22nd May 2013
Available from: http://www.ofsted.gov.uk/news/school-led-partnerships-setting-benchmark-for-high-quality-teacher-training-0 (Accessed 23/12/14).

O'Hara, M. (2014)
Teachers left to pick up pieces from cuts to youth mental health services
The Guardian, Tuesday 15 April 2014
Available from: http://www.theguardian.com/education/2014/apr/15/pupils-mental-health-cuts-services-stress-teachers (Accessed 17/4/14).

O'Neill, L., Guenette, F. & Kitchenham. A. (2010)
'Am I safe here and do you like me?' Understanding complex trauma and attachment disruption in the classroom
British Journal of Special Education, 37(4), 190–197.

Perry, B. (2006)
Applying principles of neurodevelopment to clinical work with maltreated and traumatized children
New York: The Guilford Press.

Perry, B. & Szalavitz, M. (2011)
Born for love: why empathy is essential and endangered
New York: Harper Collins

Pritzker, D. (2012)
Narrative analysis of 'hidden stories': a potential tool for teacher training
Haifa, Israel: Academic Gordon College of Education.

Riddall-Leach, S. (2003)
Managing children's behaviour
Harlow: Heinemann

Rogers, B. (2004)
How to manage children's challenging behaviour
London. Sage Publishing

Schore, A.N. (1999)
Affect regulation and the origin of the self: the neurobiology of emotional development
USA: Lawrence Erlbaum Publishing

Siegel, D. (1999)
The Developing Mind: Toward a Neurobiology of Interpersonal Experience.
New York. Guildford

Sitler, H,C. (2008)
Teaching with awareness: the hidden effects of trauma on learning
The Clearing House. Vol. 82, No. 3. Heldref Publications

Spilt, J.L. & Koomen, H.M.Y. (2009)
Widening the view on teacher-child relationships: teachers narratives concerning disruptive versus non-disruptive children
School Psychology Review, 38, 86-101

Spilt, J.L., Koomen, H.M.Y., Thijs, J.T. & Van der Leij, A. (2012)
Supporting teachers' relationships with disruptive children: the potential of relationship-focused reflection
Attachment and Human Development, 14(3), 305-318

Terr, L.C. (1991)
Childhood traumas: an outline and an overview
American Journal of Psychiatry, 148, 10-20

de Thierry, E. (2014)
Evaluating the effectiveness of a trauma training provision for teachers and their students
Manuscript in preparation.

de Thierry, E. (20 06)
The Daisy Theory
Manuscript in preparation

de Thierry, E.(2013)
The Trauma Continuum and Triangle
Manuscript in preparation

Van der Hart, O., Nijenhuis, E. & Steele, K. (2006)
The haunted self: structural dissociation and the treatment of chronic traumatisation
New York: Norton

Watkins. J.G .& Watkins, H.H. (1979)
The theory and practice of ego state therapy. In: H. Grayson (Ed.) Short term approaches to psychotherapy
New York: Human Sciences Press, pp.176-22

Watkins, J.G & Watkins, H.H. (1993)
Ego state therapy in the treatment of dissociative disorders. In: R.O. Kluft and C.G. Fine (Eds.). Clinical perspectives on multiple personality disorder
Washington DC: American Psychiatric Press, pp.277-300

Wieland, S. (2010)
Dissociation in traumatised children and adolescents
New York: Routledge

Winnicott, D.W. (1960)
The theory of the parent-infant relationship
International Journal of Psycho-Analysis, 41, 585-595

Yanowitz, K.L., Monte, E. & Tribble, J.R. (2003)
Teachers' beliefs about the effects of child abuse
Child Abuse and Neglect, 27, 483-488.

Lightning Source UK Ltd.
Milton Keynes UK
UKOW06f0434121117
312538UK00005B/270/P